ROOTED REFLECTIONS:

A Collection of Hair Stories, Trials and Triumphs

VOLUME I

Edited by
Saja Publishing Company

ROOTED REFLECTIONS:

A Collection of Hair Stories, Trials and Triumphs

Saja Publishing Company, LLC

Published in 2012 by
Saja Publishing Company, LLC.
P. O. Box 2383
Stafford, Texas 77497
www.sajapublishing.com

Printed in the United States of America.
Designed by Velin Saramov
Cover design by Jan Soriano
Cover Images courtesy of ©Shutterstock

Ordering Information: Special discounts are available on quantity purchas-
es by bookstores, wholesalers, corporations, associations, and others. For
details, contact the publisher at the address above or visit us on the web at
www.blackhairscience.com.

Publisher's Cataloging-in-Publication Data

Rooted reflections: A collection of hair stories, trials and triumphs/ edited
by Saja Publishing Company.—1st ed.
p. cm.

ISBN- 978-0-9845184-7-0 (paperback)

ISBN- 978-0-9845184-8-7 (electronic)

Library of Congress Control Number: 2012905476

" . . . BUT THE VERY HAIRS OF YOUR HEAD ARE ALL NUMBERED."

—Matthew 10:30

Contents

CONTENTS

Acknowledgments

PREPARING a book for publication takes the work, ideas and support of many, many people. We would like to personally thank the students who participated in this effort and those whose works are showcased here in these pages. Without your contribution, this book would not have been possible. We enjoyed reading your hundreds of personal essays and are honored to be able to share some of your thoughts with the world.

Aaron Miller

Marisa Williamson

Alexzander Gaither

Brittany Allen

Abia Agyekum

Jasmine Drake

Nina Goodwine

Joy Marie Sandford

Chakisha Johnson

Shaari Jenkins

Dominique Flagg

Bahareh Abhari

Melanie Ray

Tamaratare Omaya

Tatiana Flowers

Kyaunne Richardson

Nolita Pore

Aleah Carr

Tramaine Paul

Anastasia Harris

Christal Clements

Monet Abrams

Shakira Ja'nai Paye

Sabrina Walley

Charlotte Bruce

Amber May

Darian Washington

Dominique Allen

Melissa Glenn Tran-Coley

Ayres Cook

Brittany Biggett

Jace Ross

DeKeveion Glaspie

Marggy Charles

Enongo Lumumba-Kasongo

Johnene Benson

Lester Duverce

Manjit Golden

Natalia Ikheloa

Ronchelle Nelson

Cathy Ervil

Camille Bridges

Breiana Whittaker

Rebecca Webster

On Black Hair
An Introduction

E VERY single one of us has a memory about our hair. Many of us can tell our hair's *story* from our earliest days of childhood up until this very moment—and can do so with exquisite, colorful detail. When you hear these fascinating hair stories, you always find common storylines, similar themes, and recurring characters. Hair is truly a shared experience. If you listen carefully, you will even hear about the same types of hair products and appliances, almost as if we were all somehow siblings in the same home with the same mother or grandmother. Hair is also an excellent marker of time; it allows us to easily connect certain hairstyles, hair lengths and hair colors with different stages, phases and people in our lives.

Our Hair

Black or textured hair, in particular, brings with it a wide variety of emotions for the wearer over a lifetime. These feelings can range from feelings of sheer joy, love and glowing pride to feelings of fear, hate and shame in an instant. If you are reading this book now, hair has meant something to you—even in what you may believe is its unremarkable insignificance. The importance (and even lack of importance) we give our hair in our lives reveals much about how we're thinking, feeling and experiencing life. This is no novel concept; hair has always held value, even in the earliest societies. The Greeks, the Romans and our African ancestors fussed over hair just as we do today. But textured hair holds a special value. Next to our infinite range of beautiful earth skin tones, our hair is perhaps the most noticeable signifier of our *blackness*—or our connection to the black diaspora. No other type of hair has been the subject of so much attention and deliberation—both good and bad.

Our hair's history has been one fraught with unique challenges that still affect many of us—and our choices—today. Pressures from outside our community combine with pressures from within the community to create a very unique environment for personal expression through this simple appendage. Few will disagree that the average member of the black community today is probably acutely aware of even the faintest distinctions between hair textures and can quickly organize curls, coils and kinks into their various desirable and undesirable designations—an art of classification that is essentially lost on naturally straight-haired communities. It is not uncommon for even the smallest children to possess this skill for categorizing hair types and making fine distinctions such as which types of hair are preferable, which should be straightened as a matter of course, which can be worn curly as is, and so on. Many weedlike terms (i.e., *good hair, bad hair* and their cousins) have found easy root in our everyday discussions and still continue to drive a wedge between us today. The social implications surrounding our hair fibers are as complex and undeniable as the fibers' own physical bends and twists. Whole industries, counterindustries and movements have been created and resurrected to deal with black hair in all its forms.

Rightly or wrongly, the way our hair is worn and styled causes it to speak and to *suggest*, even when we are silent. For some of us, our hair is simply a cosmetic playground or accessory that we can shift and shape to suit our fancy. For others, hair becomes a gauge of one's "blackness," ethnic pride and social consciousness. The way our hair is worn or styled may even trigger particular assumptions about our sexuality, political leanings, educational level, musical tastes, worldview and personality. Books have been written, movies have been made, and billions of dollars have passed hands in an attempt to influence, control or simply understand what we do with our hair and why. Can something as simple as hair really tell us about a person's level of self-pride, the sort of music they like or how they feel about their place in this world? Perhaps . . . or perhaps not. It is a complicated subject that we simply can't resist debating.

About This Anthology

I F you were to ask me years ago about my hair, I'd tell you that it was just one of those facts of life that I wouldn't wish on my worst enemy. Today, I am absolutely in love with my hair and its ability to literally stand and command the attention of a room. But this love didn't come easily. Tears were shed, protests were made and eventually acceptance prevailed. My journey of self-discovery with my own hair led me to research the unique characteristics of this hair type and to write my first book, *The Science of Black Hair: A Comprehensive Guide to Textured Hair Care* (Amazon, $24.95). This bestselling book explores the intricacies of textured hair and offers strategies for bringing out the very best in this remarkable hair type.

As I *discovered*, I also wondered if others had ever really considered their hair and what it meant to them on a personal level. How was having textured hair today affecting people's lives? Their career choices? Self-esteem? Family relationships?

We posed this very broad question to more than five hundred students on The Science of Black Hair website (www.blackhair-science.com), and this anthology shares their responses. Why students? Because appealing to this target group allowed us to accomplish a few things at once. Many websites out there focus on beautifying individuals on the outside—but we wanted to create a unique online space with social conviction. Because our site is all about promoting healthy hair education, we also naturally support the general pursuit of education in our community as a larger social-outreach goal. In this spirit, we posed the hair question as a scholarship essay-prompt to encourage individual self-discovery and to help ease the burden of college tuition. Finally, we were simply interested in hearing what tomorrow's leaders and influencers had to say!

This anthology celebrates the reflective essays of more than forty Science of Black Hair Forum scholarship applicants who answered our question about how their textured hair has influenced various aspects of their lives. These applicants were selected for publication from a pool of more than five hundred entries. While every entrant shared an important personal experience, our review committee chose the essays contained here because of their unique voices and the diverse takes or contributions that we felt should be heard.

We encouraged each writer to reflect and speak candidly from their personal experiences, so naturally these essays represent a variety of opinions on black hair—both "popular" and "unpopular." The authors represent age groups and educational levels ranging from seventeen-year-olds to fifty-somethings and from high school seniors to Ph.D. candidates. A majority of the stories here come from writers who have not yet reached adulthood—or are only a few years into it—while others are more seasoned and have had many experiences to color their perceptions. We understand that hair means very different things to different people and at different times in our lives, and we celebrate every step of our collective and individual hair journeys. The writers, their ideas and their essays are not perfect—they're real.

We would like to commend the students who participated in this effort and extend hearty congratulations to the six scholarship winners selected this year.

This volume, we hope, is the first of many more to come. I believe very much in living the "village mentality." If it takes an entire village to raise a child, it also takes a village to support a people as well. Working together in love, we can see our community forward.

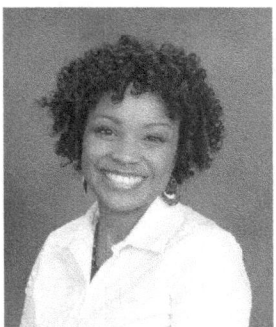

Audrey Sivasothy, author, publisher, and founder of The Science of Black Hair Forum

The Science of Black Hair Scholarship

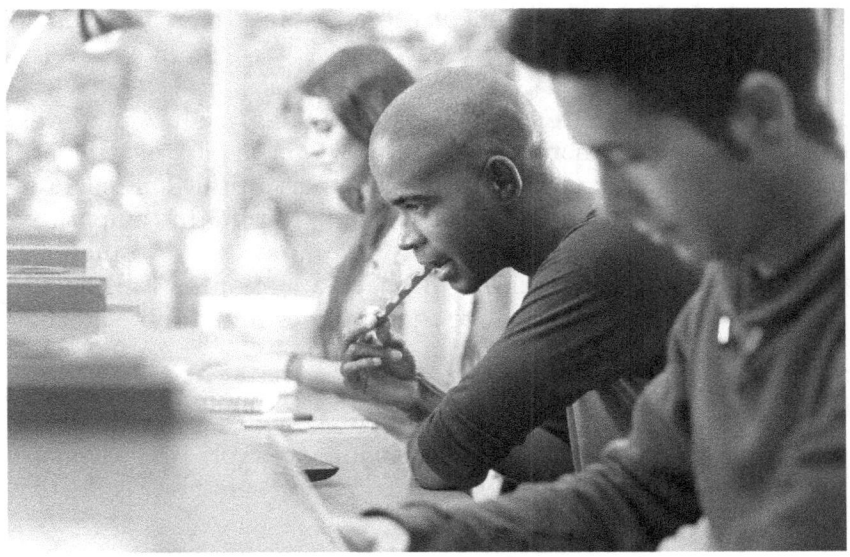

"Without education, there is no hope for our people—and without hope, our future is lost."

—Charles Hamilton Houston

T HE face of education has changed in the last fifty years. Increasingly, blacks are joining their Caucasian, Hispanic and Asian counterparts to become part of the world's educated elite. While great strides have been made in the education of black students, disparities in the attainment of higher education amongst this population continue to persist. Although the number of all college graduates has increased steadily over time, blacks and Hispanics are still less likely than whites and Asians to have completed their college education. Between black men and women, additional educational divides exist. Black women still enter and complete college at higher rates than their male peers.

These educational disparities often flow down to affect the overall earning power of blacks in the workforce. In the United States, blacks earn a percentage of the incomes of whites in similar occupations. Even among the similarly educated and across all educational levels, unemployment rates for black men and women remain disproportionately higher.

As many of us may already realize, disparities in education levels oftentimes are due not to lack of ability on the part of students, but rather to a lack of resources and opportunities for academic development. In order for black students to remain competitive in an increasingly global economy, we must strive to increase both the number of blacks in higher education as well as the number who go on to complete their studies and pursue careers and training.

Our goal at The Science of Black Hair Forum is to plant seeds of support for our members' educational endeavors with the hope that these investments will be returned to benefit our collective communities.

Our Selection Criteria

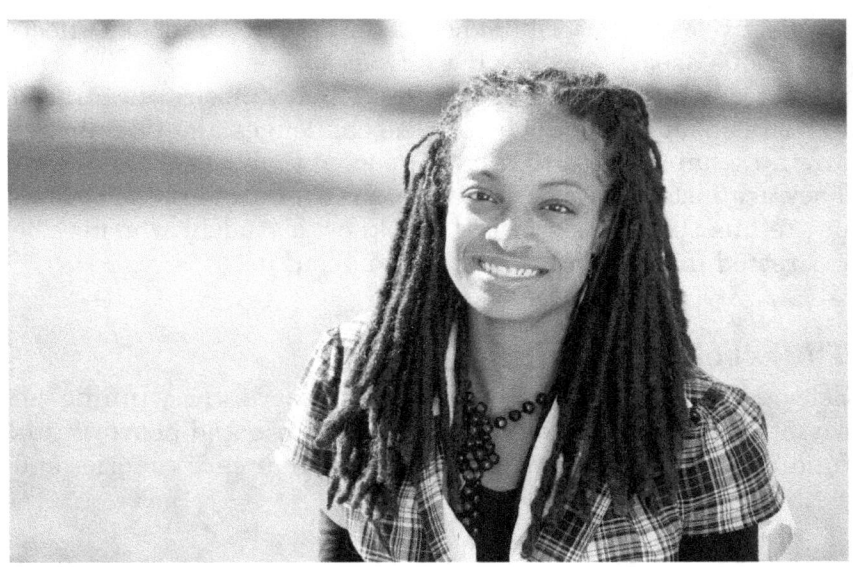

THE Science of Black Hair Forum offers annual educational awards to its member-subscribers by encouraging them to consider and reflect upon their textured hair as a driver of self-discovery. Last year, we received well over five hundred entries to our scholarship competition, and many applications were well deserving of both scholarship awards and publication. This year's scholarship Grand Prize winner received $1,000 to pursue study during the 2011-2012 school year and an invitation to be published in this year's award book. We selected a Second Prize winner to receive a $500 scholarship award and awarded four additional Honorable Mention winners prizes of $250 each toward their studies.

All scholarship opportunities sponsored by The Science of Black Hair Forum are open to students of all ages including incoming college freshmen, currently enrolled undergraduate and graduate college students, and cosmetology and technical school students. Scholarships may also be used for training courses and continuing education for career advancement in any profession. International applications are welcomed.

To apply, applicants must complete an application form and write a reflective essay describing how their textured hair has affected various aspects of their lives, from dating to career choices, self-esteem, family relationships, etc. Applicants are encouraged to write about their hair memories, challenges and triumphs—anything hair-related that has impacted their lives in any way. They are instructed to be creative, funny, serious—and to simply, tell us their hair story! If you know a student who may be interested in our program, tell them about us!

The Scholarship Winners

Selected from more than five hundred essays, the winning essay by Aaron Miller exemplified the purpose and heart of this funding effort. His essay reminds us that hair care victories and challenges know no gender.

NOTE: Essays included in this anthology have been lightly edited for space considerations, grammar and/or to simply clarify the writer's points. Every effort has been made to remain true to the writer's voice.

The Essay Collection

VOLUME I

Grand Prize Winner
Confessions of a
Hair Connoisseur

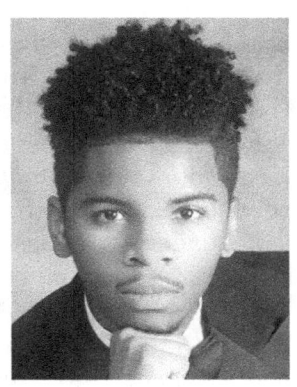

Aaron Miller
Freshman, Political Science
San Jose State University

We loved the frankness of Aaron's essay with his witty, conversational writing style. This self-proclaimed "product junkie" is addicted to leave-in conditioners and certainly provided us comic relief with his application package. He reminded us that the "hair game" knows no gender and mentioned that he can "cook, sing, dance, do hair and write." We loved it! In his "Confessions," Aaron takes us through his hair journey—from his fades, waves and texturizer-gone-wrong to his absolutely jaw-dropping, show-stopping Mohawk. He had us at hello!

SEEMS like only yesterday that I was in the bathroom with my two teenage aunts and my three brothers—Chris, Matt, and Gabe—and our aunts decided to comb each one of our heads to determine who had "the best hair." I remember how painful it was as they roughly raked the fine-toothed comb through my dry mini-Afro. After my aunts' examination, it was determined that I had the nappiest, worst hair among my brothers and me. I was only five years old. Chris was ten, Matt eight and Gabe just three. I didn't quite understand what having the worst hair meant, but it stung.

Growing up, I constantly overheard my father bragging about his hair; everybody *knew* that Gerry had that "good hair." It must have been those untraceable Irish and Indian genes every African-American claims to have "got in they family." My mother, Debra, was a licensed hairdresser who worked out of her kitchen on the side after her day job. She always kept her hair and the hair of my two sisters, Winter and Taylor,

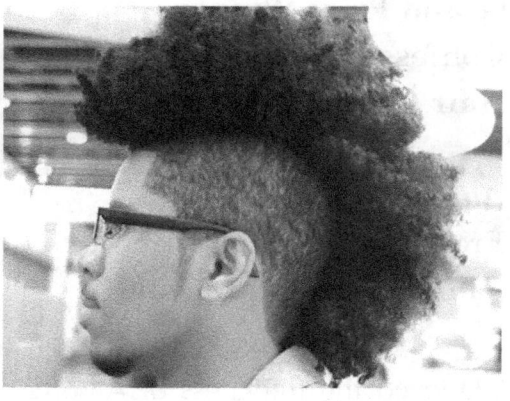

relaxed. So, for my family, when it came to talking about "good hair," the boys were the only ones up for discussion because we were the only ones with natural hair.

Let's start from the top of the hair hierarchy, shall we? Gabriel, my youngest brother, had the *best* hair; it was long, fine, smooth and curly. Matt was next: He had a curly Afro with a shiny texture. And then came Chris, who was not too far off from that. As for me, I had the supposed super-dry coily, kinky, nappy hair. Looking back, I realize that the differences between all of our hair types were so miniscule that there shouldn't even have been a discussion. But for some reason, families always feel the need to compare and organize.

As I grew up, it was just a fact, and a source of comedic relief, that AARON HAS BAD, NAPPY HAIR. I believed it, too, and so my hair was always cut very low in a fade or a taper or in waves. From kindergarten until tenth grade, I kept my hair cut short. When I was in the fourth grade, as my mom was cutting my hair she decided it was just "too nappy." She said I needed just "a little something to knock down some of the kinks." She recommended a light texturizer, but

> Looking back, I realize that the differences between all of our hair types were so miniscule that there shouldn't even have been a discussion. But for some reason, families always feel the need to compare and organize.

she used a mild relaxer. I knew relaxers made the hair straight. I didn't want that, so at first I refused. But I trusted my mom, and after some persuasive words from her, I decided to let her have her way. I remember the cool, thick cream being spread and smoothed all over my freshly cut hair—or should I say scalp?! Big no-no! That cool feeling slowly turned to tingling and then quickly into a slight burning sensation. After the whole relaxing process was complete, I looked in awe at how my new hair just lay down. I actually kind of liked the results. I did that to my hair sporadically a few more times until the fifth grade—and I reference that time period when I try to understand why relaxers become so addictive for women.

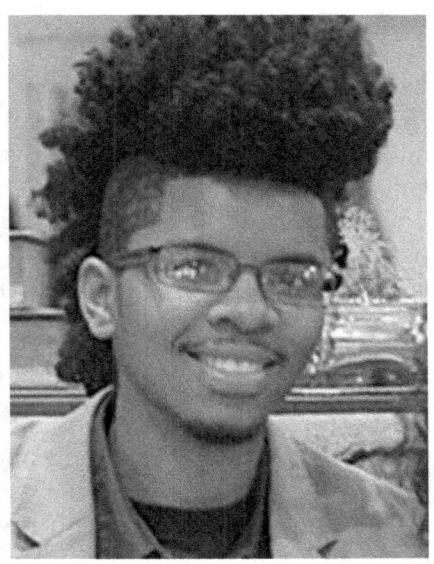

I began to cut my own hair in the fifth grade. It took some trial and error before I considered myself a formidable self-taught barber, but I got there. I found confidence and pride in cutting my own hair. None of my brothers or friends could do it. Over the next few years, until the ninth grade, I cut my hair on a regular basis and always had the same waves while my brothers had various styles. Each of them, at one point or another, had waves and cornrows, twisties, blow-outs, curly 'fros and more. I never really cared that they always were able to grow their hair out without torment and were actually encouraged to do so by our parents. I was completely content with my short hair—at least that's what I thought.

Around sophomore year, I randomly got lazy and did not cut my hair for a few weeks. I became curious about just how horrible this so-called "nappy hair" growing out of my scalp could be. So I let it grow. I remember all of my family and friends, along with my crush at the time, telling me repeatedly to "cut that stuff off!" Hearing that from my crush was especially difficult. I held off from cutting my hair for three whole months. That was a record for me. I only had about an inch and a half of hair, but I was fascinated by it. After the first stroke of the clippers, I was filled with regret and wished I had held off.

> It took some trial and error before I considered myself a formidable self-taught barber, but I got there. I found confidence and pride in cutting my own hair.

Of course everyone was happy to see it go, except for me—but I wanted to please them, so I kept it low. That summer, my crush abruptly moved away. I was devastated for a while, but life went on. Upon reflection, if that hadn't happened, I probably wouldn't have done what I was about to do. On a random day in late June 2009, I was in the bathroom cutting my hair as usual. But this time, I decided to leave the hair thicker down the middle and shorter on the sides. I did one of those little Mohawks that are popular nowadays. After I took a shower and walked out of the bathroom I was slightly nervous to see how my family would react. To my surprise, they all received it well and liked it, so I kept it for the rest of the summer.

As my junior year was rapidly approaching, I was nervous about going to registration with what, at the time, seemed like such a bold haircut. The dilemma about whether to cut it or keep it arose yet again. My mom suggested that I put a black rinse on my whole head so that my hair would not only be a richer black, but also diffuse the look of the Mohawk. I tried and liked it. I mustered up the courage to go to school with my new hair, and to my surprise, no one even noticed or mentioned it. It wasn't as noticeable as I thought it was. So, I kept my Mohawk, and it continued to grow into the school year—bigger and bigger and bigger.

During my junior year, I realized that I was not only interested in my hair, but in all hair—and in how to maintain healthy hair. I learned a lot, particularly through YouTube. The first time I grew my hair out during my sophomore year, I did not know what to do for my hair. I have curls and coils that need lots of conditioning and the proper styling products. I used a blue hair dressing (loaded with horrible petroleum), setting lotion foam and—the worst—a popular thick hair pomade during the first go-round to try to "make" my hair curly. This time, I watched countless videos and read many articles and books to gain knowledge about how to deal with my type of hair. While learning how to manage my hair, my family and I learned that my hair wasn't "bad" at all, and that it just needed some extra TLC. I became somewhat obsessed with hair and even branched out into learning about relaxed hair to help the women in my family with their hair. I've done relaxers, flatironing, curling, weave installing, roller setting, etc. I help them with it all!

As my hair continued to grow, the naysayers returned. But this time, it wasn't only negative feedback; many people actually loved my hair, and I was getting compliments left and right. I was never the most confident person as far as my appearance. I always felt that I was the unspoken worst-looking sibling. So when I started receiving compliments on a regular basis for a change, it felt extremely satisfying. I think that newfound confidence was a factor that contributed to my current relationship. My girlfriend, who is a curly girl herself, always jokes with me and says that I can never cut my hair short again because I look horrible without it.

Looking back, I realize how much having my hair has helped me grow. I have learned so much about the artistic and scientific aspects of hair. My hair has taught me how to ignore negativity and persevere in the face of adversity (that's politically correct talk for haters). Surprisingly, hair has taught me to be diligent, dedicated and determined. Trust me, sometimes those two-hour-long showers just for detangling take lots of dedication! But I cannot tell you how many people walk up to me in public just to say nice things about my once-so-called nappy hair. In my family and circle of friends I'm known as "the hair guy," and at some point in my life I'd like to go to school for hair. I never would have thought, on the day that I cut that little Mohawk, that I'd still have it two years later and be nominated for Best Hair in my school's Senior Hall of Fame. When I read that this scholarship was available, I was overjoyed. I feel that it is meant especially for me. Hair is such an important thing to me—so sharing my story while getting help to pay for San Jose State University is pure nirvana!

Scholarship Winner
The Quest for a Princess

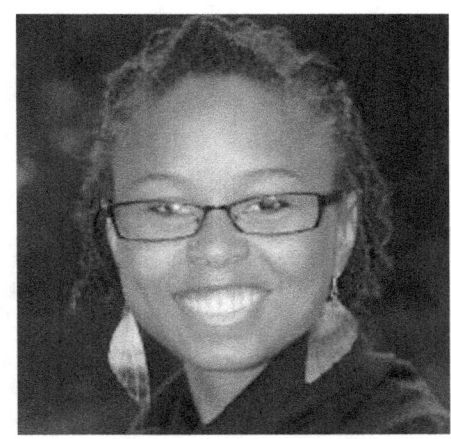

Marisa Williamson
1st Year Graduate Student,
Master of Fine Arts
California Institute of the
Arts

Marisa's interesting account of one girl's search for an "animated analogue" to call her own explains how the journey to reimagine herself led her to become an artist. Her beautifully written essay—rather poetic and dexterous in its wordplay—was a clear winner for us! We enjoyed her academic and artistic approach to her essay.

WHEN news hit the Internet several years ago that Disney would release its next animated film, *The Frog Princess*, and that that film would feature an African-American heroine, a series of posts to Harvard's black women's email list indicated that black women of a certain generation were very curious and very excited about this new addition to the coterie of Disney Princesses. Few details about the film had been released, and as a result there were many questions and speculations. A major concern—one that sparked considerable interest among my classmates—was about the creative, commercial and political resolution of the main character's hair.

The politics of black hair is hardly unexplored. In writings on the evolution of the black body in the American landscape, theorists Alice Walker and bell hooks recognize hair as a critical component of the creation and acknowledgment of self and community. The politics of hair, however, has remained relatively isolated within the black community, due in part to highly personal and

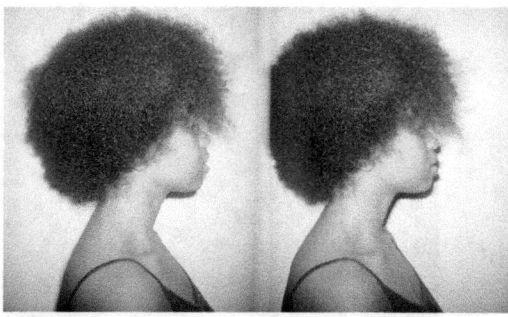

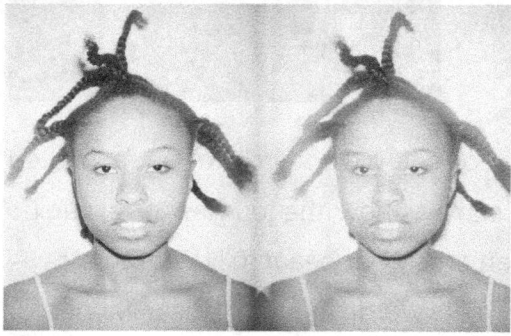

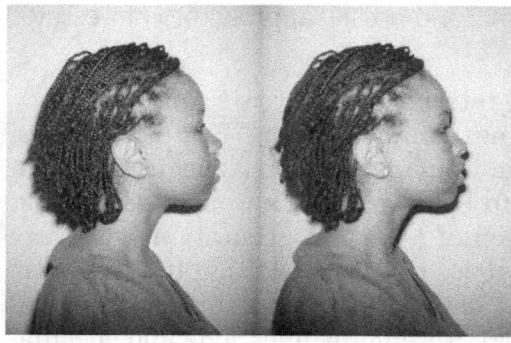

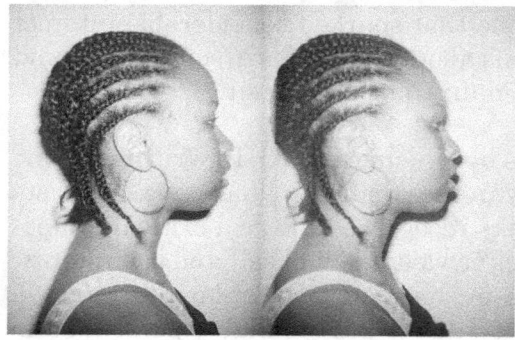

variable experiences that result in a complex, diverse and irreducible array of sentiments. There is no single ideology about black hair. There is no one way to experience black hair, just as there is no one way to be black and female in this world.

For twenty-five years, my idea of a princess has had its foundation in Disney films. I recall at age four a frantic trip with my dad to a large shopping mall in search of *The Little Mermaid*. It was a wildly popular film in 1989—and boasted a red-headed heroine who, with unprecedented speed and efficacy, empowered every ginger-haired girl in my suburban neighborhood.

When we moved to the city two years later, I embraced Belle and Jasmine as my new outlined idols. They were brave, gutsy and independent. Both wrestled with the impatience of youth and the burden of being ambitious and smart in a world in which those characteristics were valued secondarily to beauty. I saw and still do see myself in Belle. We share an interest in learning, a craving for adventure and a strong sense of obligation. While I felt my psychological identity projected and preserved on those VHS cassettes, my physical self, which was becoming quickly and awkwardly more relevant, still lacked an animated analogue.

I knew that I wasn't ugly, but I knew that I did not possess the features that made princesses beautiful. My lips were full like my dad's, my nose unusually freckled and round like my mom's. I had my paternal grandfather's peanut head and my grandmother's proud cheekbones. By fourth grade I had inherited a Jamaican booty from my mother's Jamaican mother and strong athletic thighs. My hair—nappy, first in line among my sisters to be braided by my mom on Sundays, with colorful barrettes at the end of each braid—would never grow to be long like Belle's. It would never be naturally straight like Jasmine's. It would never blow romantically along with all the colors of the wind.

> I owe the development of my deepest passions—art, imagination and education—to those youthful insecurities about hair and all that it represents.

It has been this mild but persistent dissatisfaction with reality—a sense that "what is" is not nearly as interesting as "what could be"—and the constant desire to reimagine myself and my world that has led me to be an artist. So, while I've since become much more comfortable in my skin; come to adore my hair and the myriad things I can do with it; learned to cherish my black body because it's black, beautiful and mine alone; and found a prince—or rather, a man—who is brilliant, funny, a feminist and a loving friend, I owe the development of my deepest passions—art, imagination and education—to those youthful insecurities about hair and all that it represents.

Now, as an artist, hair is a source of inspiration. It is storied, complicated, tangled and rich. Sometimes it's about assimilation—the absorption of something foreign, an incorporation of otherness.

Assimilation refers also to adaptation, resemblance, recreation and modification. To assimilate to a culture that is itself dynamic and changing is to be caught in a cycle that is at once problematic and compelling. Hair is also about process, about change over time and the malleability of image.

In my work I've traced a line of thought that follows technology, the body and nostalgia back to the public, private, physical and emotional sites where they were conceived.

Hair (a motif, a unifying strand) is in all the dusty corners, caught in the teeth of a fine-toothed comb and clustered round the drain—simultaneously and naturally central and peripheral—and often ambiguous. Hair is genetic evidence: a racial signifier or a false indicator. It is an extension, expression, suggestion of self, nothing but highly evolved fur, anything but easy, never always one thing, never always another. It is mine to render and surrender—my metaphor, my analogue, my constant variable.

> It is an extension, expression, suggestion of self, nothing but highly evolved fur, anything but easy, never always one thing, never always another. It is mine to render and surrender—my metaphor, my analogue, my constant variable.

Hair is just one way to incorporate otherness. I become stuff. Stuff becomes me. I am my hair now—as I am my shoes, my music, the movies I love, my work, my profile and my people.

Scholarship Winner
The Loc Retreat

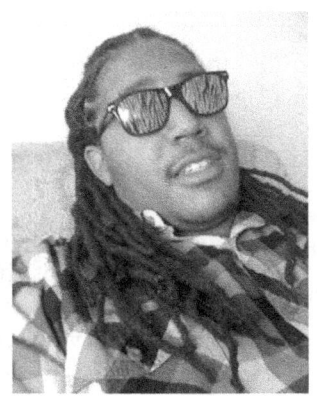

Alexzander Gaither
Senior, Music and Math
California State University,
Sacramento

Alexzander's essay about his locs is a magnificent read. At twenty-two years of age, he has not had a haircut in more than ten years. His cultivated locs, which he refers to as his "soulful antennae," were grown from a simple set of twists and have affected his work as a student of music deeply. One of the things that stands out in his essay is his dedication to his stylist. While we often scoff at those who are "chained to the chair," Alexzander paints a wonderful picture of her Sacramento retreat.

MY name is Alexzander Gaither. I'm twenty-two years old, and I haven't had a haircut since age twelve. What started as neat twists has evolved into a dedicated hair lifestyle of well-organized and cultivated forty-inch locs. The locs are an extension of both the *who* and *what* that I am. I know of no other hairstyle that could simultaneously represent my ethos and personality better. The spiritual connection with my ancestors through my hair gives me balance, strength and purpose.

My locs are soulful antennae that connect my present to my past. I feel the presence of my ancestors with each musical improvisation I play. We communicate through music. I feel the joy

> My locs are soulful antennae that connect my present to my past.

and inspiration of their creativity. Their presence grounds me and gives ancestral purpose to my academic and professional directions. I am focused.

My grandmother, Beverly Gaither, had organic locs not by selection but as a result of the depth of her many contributions under her belief that family always came first. She would never have gone into a beauty salon. From the depths of her very soul, she just could not give herself permission. Nothing was more important to her than family. She passed away when I was young, but I'll always remember the depth of her eyes, her face, her smile and her hair—a physical demonstration of just how much she loved me. I proudly shake my locs in celebration of her eternal spirit. My locs, as an essence of who and what I am, fill me with confidence because I know that I am not alone.

Keeping my locs cultivated means a two-week rotation to my stylist. She's very talented and runs a much sought-after black hair care business in Sacramento, California. Her long-term clients are faithful for a reason, and I rank among them. As she has moved around the city, I and other faithful clients have moved around with her. She's had no less than ten different business locations over the years!

> Their presence grounds me and gives ancestral purpose to my academic and professional directions. I am focused.

Thirteen years is a very long time and a considerable financial dedication to a woman who is a very important part of my persona. We've been together from the very beginning. She gave me a discount in those early days because I once told her that I attended high school and college simultaneously. She didn't believe me and challenged me to prove it. When I showed her my grades, she gave this brotha a break until I graduated from high school.

Her salon today is an immersion in complete trust and relaxation. The reception area is Afro-centric, aroma and music therapeutic, and comfortable. Even for a big brotha such as myself. Many of her customers have been with her for so long that she no longer accepts new customers. My hair is a showcase of her many hair care talents.

But don't misunderstand me—her salon is a well-oiled machine, and unannounced cancellations will cost you! She works Monday to Saturday from 7 A.M. to 9 P.M. She does not play about with her schedule. To miss your appointment is to take a trip to the end of the line and another two-week wait. Failure to pay is automatic grounds for ejection from her calendar and reason to lose sleep. You can be late if you want to be, but in her world, early is on time, and on time is late! When a client's time allotment is up, it's all about the rise and fly. I've heard "Be on time next time" before.

> I'll always remember the depth of her eyes, her face, her smile and her hair—a physical demonstration of just how much she loved me.

My scalp wouldn't survive an entire month without her touch, so I haven't missed an appointment for several years now. When LaShawn at Head Turners gets to scraping and massaging my scalp, it's almost like heavy petting. It's all a brotha can do to keep from moaning out loud. She knows I'm appreciating, so she always schedules additional time to give my scalp the once and twice over with those magical fingers of hers.

In conclusion, I can't imagine wearing my hair in any other style. I'm not certain as to when, if ever, I'll change my hairstyle, but if I do, it will be for some really important reason. My locs are as much a part of me as I am a part of them. They connect me to and remind me of the strength of my ancestors, who fill me up with their pride and well wishes to see me complete my education and become professionally successful. I shake my locs wildly in celebration of their many contributions and give thanks and praise to them for giving me the opportunity to share in the continuum of their combined spiritual energy.

Scholarship Winner
Fly

Brittany Allen
1st year Masters in Public
Health
George Washington
University

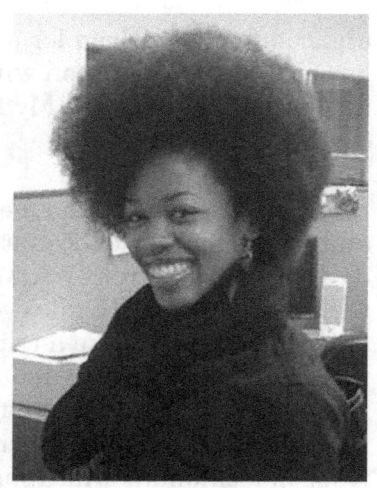

Brittany's essay was another one of our fast favorites. Her opening words? "I'm so fly." And . . . she definitely is! Her essay is very personal, and her writing style is in your face and edgy. It's different, and we liked it! Her essay describes the versatility of her hair, how her Afro drew her last boyfriend to her, and how she has learned to "own" her look. Her hair pride pours through her pages.

"I'M *so fly!*"

I love my 'fro! It's big, it's bodacious, it's beautiful, it's amazing. According to my grandmother, it's a sign of royalty.

"Don't cut your hair," she told me. "It's your crowning glory."

And it is!

Anyone can look at a 'fro, and whether it's big and perfectly rounded or lopsided or unkempt, it will always tend to look like a crown. My 'fro is soft. I've been told it looks like a big, fluffy pillow. My hair is versatile. I can wear two-strand twists, cornrows, straw curls or, if I so choose, straighten it out into a perfectly layered wrap. One of my friends always jokingly says, "I wonder what's next in Brittany's three hundred and sixty-five days of hairstyles?" My hair is fashionable and trendsetting. Hollywood is finally seeing the true beauty in tightly coiled hair like mine, celebrating the looks of Erykah Badu, Corrine Bailey Rae and Angie Stone.

> Anyone can look at a 'fro, and whether it's big and perfectly rounded or lopsided or unkempt, it will always tend to look like a crown.

"All the boys die, when I walk by with my Afro puff!"

My 'fro drew my last boyfriend to me. I was sitting at a table with beautiful black women who were wearing locks, weaves and relaxers. I was the only one wearing a 'fro, and he noticed me! His first words were, "How did you get your hair like that? You are so gorgeous!" It was love at first sight! I find it a bit ironic that so many sisters believe that long, straight hair is more attractive than our natural hair. When I talk to many brothers, I find that more of them prefer natural hair over relaxed hair and weaves.

So many people admire natural hair. My coworkers constantly make comments like, "Wow, one day it looks like it's an inch long, and the next day it's huge." Some even reach over to touch it, but we all know that's a no-no. Surprisingly, I get a lot of comments from older people as well. They tell me I remind them of their high school and college days in the 1960s and 1970s. I get nicknames like Soul Sistah, Angela Davis, Lauryn Hill and (my favorite) Foxy Brown. It's encouraging to be compared to such powerful and strong women.

"I'm so tough!"

My hair is strong. I can do whatever I want to it, and as long as I keep it properly moisturized, it will not break. It is made of a protein called keratin and contains melanin (eumelanin to be exact), which provides its color and adds incomparable strength. My hair is sometimes called kinky, sometimes nappy. Some people are offended by the term *nappy*, but I'm not. When I think of nappy hair, I think of hair that is rebellious, resistant and rambunctious. It makes its own rules and does what it wants. Each strand can be stretched from root to tip, and with its release— boing!—it springs back into its intricate curly state. My hair can be dyed to any color in a box of Crayolas, from Canary Yellow to Tumbleweed to Raw Sienna.

My hair is high maintenance. It requires moisture replenishing each time I shampoo and condition, to avoid breakage. My hair loves the combination of pure shea butter and the ever-so-fragrant Kemi-Oyl. My hair demands high-quality products. It demands the best. And it deserves it.

"Back it up!"

My hair was first relaxed when I was six. Usually I wore my hair in simple styles like curls or wraps. Besides getting kinky twists a few times, I never wore weaves or braids. I decided to go natural after I let a friend color my hair—bright red, to be exact— and it broke off badly. I decided to just chop it all off instead of trying to repair the damaged hair while waiting for the rest to grow back. Since then, I have not looked back! My stylist had been doing my hair for thirteen years and offered to continue relaxing it in a new, shorter style— because she did not know how to do natural hair. To both her and my mother's dismay, I politely declined. I decided to wear an itty-bitty 'fro and watch it grow!

> Some people are offended by the term nappy, but I'm not. When I think of nappy hair, I think of hair that is rebellious, resistant and rambunctious. It makes its own rules and does what it wants.

"You can't get next to me with my Afro puff!"

Natural-haired beauties are viewed differently among African-American women. We are seen as nonconformists and politically involved fighters. At other times we are perceived as earthy neo-Soul lovers and organics. These are stereotypes, but different perspectives do hold true for different people. Personally, I've always seen myself as a nonconformist. I never really felt like I fit in with a lot of people my age. I do care for the earth, and I enjoy neo-Soul music—but I've never been into politics, and I'm slow to fight. I have always been a bit shy, but cutting my hair, as simple an action as it seems, really did make me tough. I get a lot of compliments now because I've learned to own my look, but when I first cut my hair, I faced disapproval from a lot of people—most significantly my mother. She hated the fact that I cut all of my hair off and didn't talk to me for a while after I did it. Learning to love my look despite what she and others said made me courageous, confident and strong. And looking at a young lady with a big, bodacious 'fro, what else would you expect?

"I'm so fly!
All the boys die, when I walk by with my Afro puff!
I'm so tough!
Back it up!
You can't get next to me with my Afro puff!"

Scholarship Winner
Papa's Schoolgirl

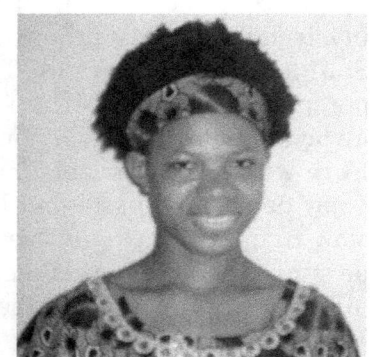

Abia Agyekum
Junior, Biology
Oakwood University

Abia's essay gave the reviewers a taste of her Ghanaian culture. In her family's tradition, short-cropped cuts for girls are the gold standard that present to society the portrait of a serious, well-groomed student. Abia chronicles her stand of momentary defiance in her essay, and it leads to an interesting outcome. We loved this essay!

D OES hair make a woman?

I was born in Ghana, West Africa. For young students in Ghana, our short-cropped haircuts represent educational opportunity. In Africa, not even primary school is free, so our uniforms and hair announce that our parents can afford to school us. At most schools in Africa, a cropped haircut is required for both girls and boys. But in general, short styles are part of our culture. They are less expensive to maintain, and in our always-hot climate, cropping short is an efficient way of keeping cool.

Well, that was fine in Ghana! When my Papa brought me to America in 2005, he informed me of his mandate about my hair. He decreed:

"You will wear your hair in African style, until high school is finished."

Not having a vote, I was comfortable with it. As the end of sophomore year approached, Papa informed me that I could grow my hair until it was time for fall term. I thought, Great! My hair is naturally very thick (from him) and reddish. This would be the first time in my life that I would be allowed to grow my hair. My hair grew fast over the summer months, and my Aunt Jerrie took me to get my first and only perm treatment at age sixteen. Well, when the beautician finished, I could not believe that *my hair* was so long, soft and beautiful. It was lovelier than I could have ever imagined. I proudly wore my new coiffure for more than a month. Did I mention that I didn't mind all the looks and compliments coming my way? Too soon summer was ending, and I conveniently forgot about the hair condition Papa had set.

"Doctor," Papa reminded me, using his name for me, *"time to get your hair cut!"*

Reality can be so cruel. With my new hair, I had invented a new me—or so I thought. A me that was Americanized, yeah, a me that heard what my mates had been saying:

"Girl, you have rights! He can't make you cut your hair if you don't want to."

What they were saying was what I wanted to hear. The only issue was: Papa is a very stubborn African man. In Africa, a father's word is final and not often to be challenged. We were in America now, but Papa didn't get that memo. For him, school was serious business, and it was time to look like a student again. I begged, but he wouldn't budge! I pouted; he ignored me. His only focus and demand was:

> With my new hair, I had invented a new me—or so I thought. A me that was Americanized, yeah, a me that heard what my mates had been saying:
>
> "Girl, you have rights! He can't make you cut your hair if you don't want to."

"It's time to cut your hair."

Cut my long, beautiful red locks that had taken me all of six weeks to grow? He must be crazy! Doesn't he see how good I look to everyone?

For the first time in my life, I refused his directive.

I waited and looked for the angel Gabriel because I knew my life would end. But, somehow, I was alive. I had refused to cut my hair, and I was still breathing. I savored life for a few moments. But Papa's mind had not changed. As he told me what I would do, I blurted out something and headed for the door. I decided to run away rather than cut my hair. I had no money and no plan. This was a spontaneous move, and I had no idea where to go or what to do—but I felt empowered.

I walked five miles and sat in the park. Would you believe, he didn't even attempt to come after me? What a turkey! I spent the whole day in the park, forgetting that night would come. As night came, I was tired and hungry—but I still had my hair. Foolishly, I spent the night in the park. When day came, I didn't feel good at all about my stand—but I still had my hair. *Onyonkopon*—God—laid on His hand and protected me until some friends saw me and took me home with them.

Four days passed, and Papa still had not looked for me. (I told you that he is stubborn!) I still had my hair, but now I was wondering if it was worth it. All my life, Papa had always told me I was *mi c'obaa cocoa fefefe*: his beautiful red girl. Now, in this predicament, I didn't feel beautiful at all—but I still had my hair.

Finally, I called home and asked if I could come.

Papa's response was:

"Is your hair cut?"

"Not yet," I said in a tearful small voice.

"If you are ready to cut it properly for school, come."

I went home, and he cut my beautiful long hair short. Very short.

The strangest thing happened after he was finished. As I looked into his eyes, I could see how much he loved me. After I had eaten, showered and oiled my African-schoolgirl-style head, I had never felt more beautiful.

Does hair make a woman?

Not this one!

Scholarship Winner
One Giant Leap for Mankind

Jasmine Drake
Junior, Biology
University of Virginia

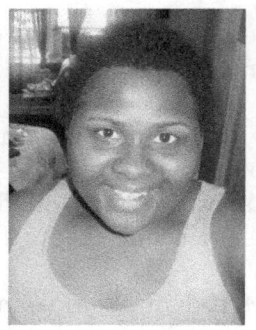

Jasmine's essay certainly stood out from the pack. Her boldness is as clear as her baldness as she describes her decision to shave head to raise money for childhood cancer research. Her ability to make what some of us would deem the ultimate beauty sacrifice to be a blessing to others is admirable. While many of us ask or wonder whether or not our hair defines us, Jasmine lives her answer. She is certainly *not* her hair—and all the more beautiful for it.

"Y OU look so pretty" were the words my best friend told me as we saw my hair on the floor. On March 24, 2011, I decided to have all of my hair shaved off to raise money for pediatric cancer research at a St. Baldrick's Foundation event. For five months, I had pondered whether my hair should be shaved off. The constant predictions I had as to what others would say about me filled me with anxiety and worry during the final days leading up to the event. *Would people think I look ugly? Would I lose some of my respect?* All of these questions were in my mind at the St. Baldrick's event.

After my moment of hair loss, I realized that my fear of losing my hair was an illusion of doubt. I did not think I could pull off a bald look—but I did, and this was a huge accomplishment for me. Through my hair triumph, I realized that hair does not define me. Hair is only a component that can easily perish. The internal factors that constitute who I am are far more important and are forever ingrained in me.

As an African-American, I deal with the stigma surrounding our hair on a daily basis. In my middle school and high school, the majority of African-American females relaxed their hair because they wanted to look and feel pretty. I was one of them, letting society tell me how I should look. The media promotes advertisements of African-Americans sporting straight hair, disseminating the message that straight hair makes a woman beautiful. Well, this "beauty" was damaging to my hair. I had many split ends, my hair smelled of a hot curling iron when I washed it, and the money necessary to keep my hair straight was financially burdensome to me. I thought that if I went natural, then my hair would be healthier, and I would still look beautiful to people in my high school.

My decision to go natural in 2008 did not solve my healthy hair problem or resolve my desire to straighten my hair. Although I enjoyed having curly hair at times, I continuously altered it, breaking the chemical bonds of my hair strands with heat and transforming them into straight, thin strands of hair. Once I went natural, it took twice the effort to make my hair straight again. As much as I tried to work with my curly hair, society loved my straight hair. I did not think that I was beautiful unless my hair was straight. Once I realized that my natural hair journey was not the solution to my self-esteem issues, I decided to participate in St. Baldrick's and found my solution to conquering my hair problems.

> As an African-American, I deal with the stigma surrounding our hair on a daily basis.

Cutting my hair off was the most enriching experience for me. Even though my best friend told me that I looked pretty, the most important thing was that I finally felt pretty. Once I touched my naked scalp in the forty-degree weather of Charlottesville, Virginia, no stigma could affect how I felt about myself. I am very happy I have no hair because I finally have control over how I define myself. I *feel* beautiful because of what I did for people with cancer. When I walk outside, I do not worry about whether or not a person thinks I am ugly because I *know* I am beautiful. My courage to cut all my hair off for people with cancer is

> I am very happy I have no hair because I finally have control over how I define myself. I feel beautiful because of what I did for people with cancer.

beautiful. My personality, my knowledge and all of the internal components that make up who I am are beautiful. As an African-American, the hair stigma no longer affects me, because I do not let hair define who I am; I define who I am.

A Journey There and Back

Nina Goodwine

N o one could believe it. In class, at lunch and in the hallways, they looked at me as if I had just beamed down from Jupiter. They were surprised, worried, humored:

"I would never have the guts to do that!"

"Oh my gosh, Nina! Did you have cancer?"

The band director was the meanest. The office called for me over the P.A., and in his typical lame-comedian style, he said in front of the entire class, "I hope they have the rest of her hair up there."

Some kids laughed. Some were stunned. I just trudged up to the office, head down, silent.

That was my first natural-hair experience, at age thirteen.

The band director apologized profusely after my mom called the school, but the damage, literally, had already been done. After tight braids, bad relaxers and habitual picking, my hair needed an extreme makeover. So my dad took me to the barbershop over the summer and they shaved my hair to about half an inch. My enormous forehead—and my insecurities—surfaced. I had friends, but I was terribly shy and hated my round body and the rash my glasses left on my face. My mother always told me I was beautiful, but I didn't believe her. All I wanted were a boyfriend, a fan base and the white-girl pendulum ponytail. If I had any chance of becoming pretty and popular, the baldy killed it.

Any black woman will tell you that a girl's hair defines her self-image early and brings her both joy and pain for years. When I was in elementary school, my grandmother and I would sit in front of a stove with Blue Magic grease and a hot comb so she could press my hair. She'd set the comb on the eye, wipe it with a paper towel to make sure it wasn't too hot and sizzle my hair from the scalp down to the ends. The straightening would burn my ears sometimes, but that was part of the beautification process. While humming hymns, she would adorn twisted plaits with bright barrettes and baubles. I'd thank her when she finished, but she'd shake her head." Don't thank me," she'd insist. "Just say, 'Grow more hair.'" And with her care, it seemed that I could. Although the grease stains on the school-bus seats weren't cute, fresh plaits always made me feel like I had great hair.

> All I wanted were a boyfriend, a fan base and the white-girl pendulum ponytail.

But after my stepmom slapped a rotten-egg-smelling, tender-scalp-burning, mother-enraging relaxer on my head to make my ten-year-old hair more "manageable," a series of unfortunate hair days—okay, years—fell on me. And let me tell you, kids in Gulfport, Mississippi, didn't play in the nineties. If your hair was nappy, your jeans had detergent stains on them or your breath smelled a little . . . fragrant, they'd never stop teasing you. Adults weren't exempt, either. 'Tween boys serenaded me with the "Just For Meeeee" kiddie relaxer anthem when I'd walk down the hall. "Ole water-head girl" and "five-head" were also crowd favorites. They teased me from middle school to tenth grade.

After myriad hairstyles, a ton of humiliation and high school graduation, I moved north to attend Howard University in Washington, D.C., where black girls had some of the longest, prettiest hair I'd ever seen. My hair was so straight from years of relaxers that my ends were translucent and perpetually shoulder-length, so it was time for another makeover. Fortunately, my older hair-stylist sister, who had moved to Maryland before I did, put me on a recovery plan that didn't, for the most part, include hecklers. With weaves and only two relaxers a year (instead of about eight), she whipped my hair into incredible shape. It was winter 2007, and I was so eager to see my progress that I took my weave out, got a relaxer and hit the floor. The year I'd turn twenty-one, my wildest hair dream was real—soft, straight hair down my back. All mine . . . and gorgeous. I curled it. I rolled it. It bounced. It swung. I felt pretty. Men liked it. Ministers touched it at altar call. I was in heaven.

But I couldn't stay.

In Gulfport, "freezing" was somewhere in the forties. I didn't even know how to tie a scarf before I moved to Maryland. During Christmas vacations, I'd visited my mother and survived a few snowstorms, but I didn't realize how vicious Northeastern winters are on the integumentary system: crocodile legs, crusty feet—and split ends. My sister kept trimming those ends, but it didn't matter. I was split pea soup and furious. Years of growth and progress were futile. I seethed. I smoldered. But I wasn't patient enough to start over. After I chopped my hair into a swishy bob, I started twisting it with gel to mimic the kinks that grow naturally from my head. I volleyed between weaves and the pseudonatural look before my younger sister, who's also a hairstylist, hacked it all off the day after Christmas. And there I was again. *Completely exposed.* But this time, I wanted to be.

> The year I'd turn twenty-one, my wildest hair dream was real—soft, straight hair down my back. All mine . . . and gorgeous. I curled it. I rolled it. It bounced. It swung. I felt pretty. Men liked it. Ministers touched it at altar call. I was in heaven.

I moved to the front lines of the war on relaxer, the "creamy crack." With my tiny coils, I pitied girls with long, straight hair. While the "system" had conned them into thinking they were more beautiful processed, my hypnosis had worn off, and I felt I was better for it. No matter how militant I tried to be, though, I didn't feel good. I couldn't get any guy's attention—at least not that of the ones I found attractive. I hated going to the bathroom before class to fix the mess my winter hat had squashed, and I hated wearing hair bands and the pain in my arms from twisting my strands every night. I fled back to the weaves.

Some women know how to rock their kinks. Starlets like Chrisette Michele, Solange Knowles and countless women on the streets of D.C. and elsewhere prove this every day. But I've tried it, and despite my every intention to fearlessly embrace my raw self, I'm not comfortable wearing my hair natural right now. The short natural's relatively simple upkeep tempts me, but I've decided to admire from afar. And I'm learning, thankfully, that that's okay. I may go natural again someday, but I dared myself instead to remove the weave and rock a super-short, relaxed cut with choppy layers at the crown. It's been a revelation—maintenance is virtually nonexistent, save for a bit of pomade on the sides and tips to give the style sheen and dimension. Washing, blowdrying and setting it takes all of twenty minutes, and a paper wrap and silk scarf keep it tight overnight. I love how my haircut makes everything in my wardrobe cooler, and the compliments I've received are icing on the cake. I have to keep it trimmed and relaxed, but when I look at my hair every day, I wonder how I wore any other style.

Your hair should be one way you express your individuality, regardless of what your family, friends, the media or random men you're not interested in say. I think it's better to wear a hairstyle you're comfortable with than to shave or straighten your hair to assert your "blackness" or appease a nap-leery mainstream. I've made peace with these playful dark-brown coils in a way that works for my personality, my lifestyle and my taste. After a years-long tussle with my locks, that acceptance is the best gift I could give myself.

Teaching Ms. Johnson and the Brothers

Joy Marie Sandford

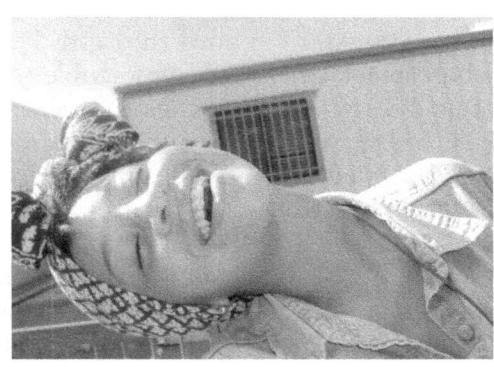

A ND she told us we looked crazy.

Couldn't believe it. *Ms. Johnson.*

Ms. Ain't-Too-Proud-to-Bring-My-Cane-to-Work Johnson . . . Ms. "How Ya'll Doin'" Johnson . . . parka-in-seventy-one-degree-weather Ms. Johnson.

Ms. Johnson was "just looking out for us" when she politely told my best friend and me—surrounded, mind you, by about nine doe-eyed freshmen who had just finished complimenting us on our style—that we looked a hot mess. Now, I know the end of the day isn't the best time to catch any naptural chick like my-self, but sheesh! *A hot mess?* "I love what you all are doin' wit da natural look and all, but—yeah, I cain't git down wit *' dis*," she winced, sweeping two fingers back and forth between the tufts of black and dirty blond that belonged to my friend and me. I choked down hurt breaths with, "Sth, Ms. Johnson, you so crazy" as best I could before my smile went limp and wormy. My natural scared her into a bold enunciation of her disapproval that only a woman of her age and wisdom could get away with.

> My natural scared her into a bold enunciation of her dis-approval that only a wom-an of her age and wisdom could get away with. I could only imagine the voices in the heads of the not-so-bold.

I could only imagine the voices in the heads of the not-so-bold. Scary thought.

They didn't all hate them: my goldish, supple wind curls. As a matter of fact, the majority loved them, applauded them, beamed toothy smiles at me on my way to the bathroom. "Love your hair!"

they said. And I'm sure they did. I was and still am in a place where black girls feel comfortable praising one another—most of us do, anyway. And the other-skinned girls felt the same. My best friend and I, with our natural hair and natural smiles, felt loved. We felt real. And despite the interference Ms. Johnson felt necessary to throw, we felt free. But we were lonely.

"We" is Asha, my best friend since the fifth grade, and me. We speak a language that the people around us have only an ear for. We speak to each other with words best described by that ticklish phenomenon that burns in the throats of other people when they catch a crumb of our conversation. That tip-of-the-tongue rhythm sort of buzzes between the two of us while onlookers and listeners smirk quizzically, with eyes squinted." What are you guys talking about?" they quip, when really they mean, "What was that? Say that again. I've heard that before. I've felt this before." And we just nod like nice girls and carry on. We know we're not the norm, but we hoped that by now, someone would appreciate us. *Someone of the male variety.*

"When are you going to take them out?"

"Um, not any time soon. Maybe like four, five years."

This was the third time my friend guy asked me about my locs. I turned my wind curls to locs about eight months ago, and every month since, a friend guy of mine felt the need to bring them up. But this—this was this particular friend guy's third time asking. The first time I laughed, hoping he was joking: "Ha, ha. Very funny, Henry. Anyway. . . ." But I knew he was serious. He wasn't the first boy to ask me about my plans for "prettier" hair. When he started to badger, probably the second or third of my friend guys to do so, I knew my brothers had a problem with it. Asha and I have exhausted the conversation of why it is black boys don't want us. *I thought they liked different girls?* We're tired of talking about it. Tired and dissatisfied. But even in our fatigue, having to face the music—that no matter the nerve, the dynamism we exude via style, attitude or otherwise, they don't like our kind—I think would be more detrimental to us than continuing our quest for the straight answer that doesn't exist. Detrimental to our spirits, our vigor in backing this stand against the façade of beauty that is so frequently embraced by my sisters, young and old. Detrimental to our self-esteem, really.

So, rather than give in and admit our insignificance in the eyes of the brothers we so badly want (I mean *badly*), we question their actions like confused, exasperated mothers. We shrug off silly "When you gone git yo' hair done" questions, and excuse the harassing fingers of misunderstood, misguided peers who find curious our locs and wind curls. We just deal. And perhaps as we mature, so will our understanding of who we are in the context of our culture, and so will our resilience in the wake of rejection, and so will our self-embrace. Who knows? My brothers might someday love these locs and wind curls, might want to play in them like the freshmen do. But until that day comes, I'll love them, play with them, style and smile at them because they are in me, and I am in them. It's all right if these boys are blind; even if the world doesn't see me, it's all good. I see me.

> But I knew he was serious. He wasn't the first boy to ask me about my plans for "prettier" hair.

No Chemistry Required
Chakisha Johnson

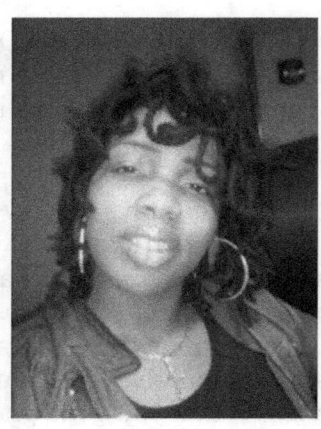

MY mother was a praying woman. As such, prior to her death in 1996, she often saw fit to pray about one subject in particular: my hair. With eyes closed and hands stretched upon my adolescent head, my mother petitioned the Creator to "heal the naps" (as if my kinky hair were an ailment). Going so far as to anoint my head with oil, my mother was sure to remind me that I inherited my hair from my father's side of the family, laying no claim to my coarse tresses. Jokingly said in love, there was undoubtedly seriousness in her requests.

As a child, my mother's petitions were anything *but* funny. In hindsight, however, I must admit that her unorthodox prayers were hilarious. Able to see the bright side in most anything nowadays, I recognize these events for both their comedic and their degrading attributes.

Hair is perhaps the most important aspect of physical appearance. A source of pride, shame or any variation of the two, hair plays a vital role in people's lives. I know firsthand the pleasures and pains associated with hair. Born and raised in Washington, D.C., my hair gives testimony to my African heritage. I have coarse (a.k.a. nappy) hair. Never a problem for me in my own opinion, it was the opinions of others that tried to persuade me to hate my hair and consequently myself. Many thought it strange of me to *want* to wear my hair in its natural state when I was younger, at a time

> My mother was a praying woman.
>
> . . .
>
> She often saw fit to pray about one subject in particular: my hair.

when Black Pride was not in vogue. Like so many of my peers, I was often forced to get a perm because nappy just wasn't an acceptable presentation in my house. Far from simple grooming and upkeep standards, what this taught me was that I wasn't acceptable in my natural state.

This message that straight is best (the "good hair" syndrome, as I call it) was a resounding message heard not only in my family, but also in my neighborhood, in magazines, on T.V. and through other media. Fast-forward one generation ahead: While natural textures are seemingly more appreciated, the "good hair" syndrome is still very much alive and well in the black community.

If I had a dollar for every time I've heard a black person use the phrase "good hair" while referring to a fine texture, I would be funding this scholarship myself! Stemming from slavery, there has been a sense of self-hatred embedded in the minds of black people, and many refuse to let go of these degrading ideas. Straight hair is NOT BETTER than kinky hair; neither is kinky hair better than straight! It's a notion so farfetched to so many that it hurts my heart. What many fail to realize is that if there is to be something *good*, by default, there must be something *bad* to counteract that good thing. So . . . if straight is good, this tells me that coarse is therefore bad.

It's taken me a long time to truly be content with myself and my hair, but I've made it to that "Black (and everything associated with it) Is Beautiful" promised land. I LOVE my nappy hair! I really do! I never have to run from the rain in fear of water disturbing a perm; neither do I have to alter myself to accept myself. I'm perfectly perfect just the way God made me. I only wish there were more of my people who felt this way.

> What many fail to realize is that if there is to be something *good*, by default, there must be something *bad* to counteract that good thing

Today, I have lovely locks. I've been completely natural for thirteen years, and I've rocked everything from a bush to braids to a feminine Caesar—and I get plenty of kudos (not to mention looks from men). I stand out just by being me. While there are times when accentuating our natural beauty is warranted, changing our hair from its natural state to a chemically altered state all in the name of beauty is not a must. If we as black women and men choose to do this, this is okay . . . so long as we acknowledge that the science of black hair requires no chemistry!

Standing Tall
Shaari Jenkins

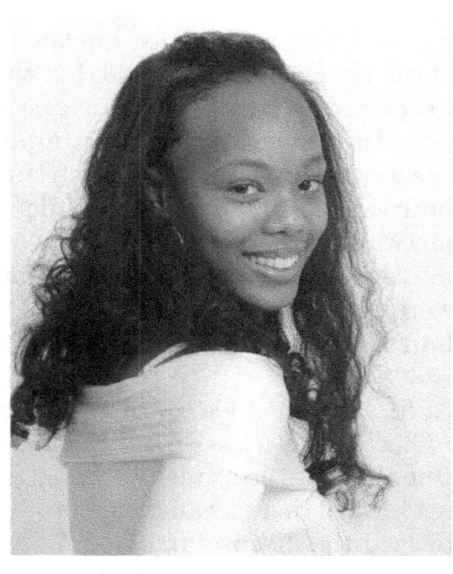

WHEN I was a little girl, my hair used to be the physical attribute for which I was known. People used to compliment me on how long my hair was and ask my mom where I got it done. As I got older, women on the street would ask me, "Is your hair a weave" or "What kind of hair is that?" When I got asked those questions, it never bothered me. If anything, I would laugh.

A few years ago, my hair story changed. One day when my mom was putting my hair in rollers, she noticed spots on my head that were without hair. She didn't panic, but I did. At first, we thought the spots were the result of a lack of vitamins. My mom made sure that I took my vitamin supplements regularly, and the spots slowly started to grow hair. I thought that was the end of that, but it wasn't. A year later, I was getting ready for prom, and the spots where back, only this time it was worse. I had to make sure my hair covered the spots because I didn't want anyone to see them.

My mother took me to the dermatologist, and I was diagnosed with the autoimmune disease alopecia areata. To sum it up, I have patches (spots) on my scalp that have no hair. They can be the size of a quarter or even bigger. They can grow back, but seeing new growth can take up to a year. (Thankfully, all of the bare spots I've had have been in

> When I was a little girl, my hair used to be the physical attribute for which I was known.

places where they can be hidden by the rest of my hair.) I did all of the research that I could, but the more I researched, the more I became discouraged: no cure, no reason for occurrence. I felt defeated and ugly. My hair was thinning out while my eyelashes and eyebrows were falling out. My friends and family would say, "Your hair looks different. Have you done something new? You've been plucking your eyebrows, haven't you?" Comments like those would make matters worse. It only meant that the effects of the disease were obvious to others. Of course, I wouldn't tell anyone why my hair looked different; I was afraid of being judged or glanced at.

At first, my attitude toward all of this was, *That's alright. At least I finally know what's wrong with me. It should get better over time.* But that attitude quickly changed. I became bitter, angry even, not toward those around me but toward the disease and God. I would frequently cry myself to sleep, hoping that when I woke up, it would all just be a bad dream. Thinking about my future always scared me. I would say to myself, *What if go bald? People will know if I wear a wig.*

> I did all of the research that I could, but the more I researched, the more I became discouraged: no cure, no reason for occurrence.

Will anyone be able to love me? Who would be attracted to a girl that looks like this? I prayed—really prayed—for God to heal me, but nothing really changed. I was still losing my hair, and nothing could be done about it. *Why? Why me God? Why this? What did I do?*

To this day, I still don't know the answer, and I probably won't know anytime soon, but I'm not bitter or angry anymore. There are moments when I become sad or cry a little because I wish it would go away, but I don't cry nearly as much as I used to. There is no use in getting myself worked up over something that I cannot control or fix. Thinking about the positive aspects of this disease helps me on the hard days. I'm thankful that I still have hair, that even though the spots are large, they aren't visible to others and that those whom I have told still see me for myself. It almost seems ridiculous to complain. Even though my hair was my "defining attribute" when I was younger, it doesn't define who I am today. It's just hair; I will still be me, with or without it.

On Balancing Creativity and Professionalism
Dominique Flagg

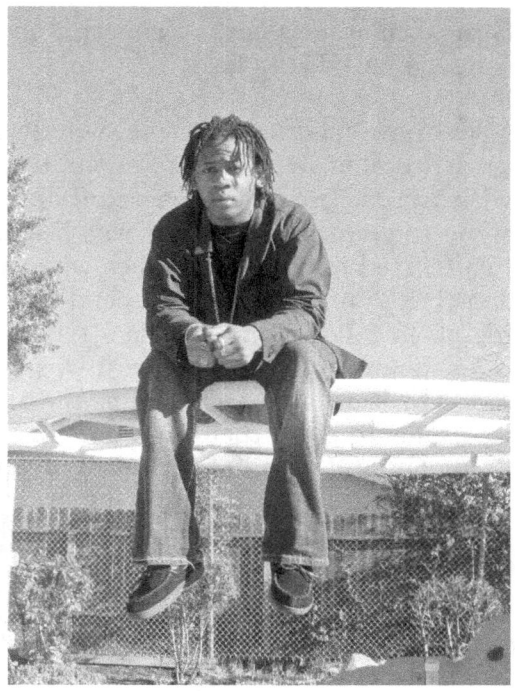

Growing up the son and nephew of hairstylists—black hair was all I knew. Every day I got out of school and walked to the shop where my mom and aunts worked for countless hours until one of them was off to finally go home.

It is safe to say that when it came to hair, I was indirectly educated. Geographically, my closest cousins were all girls, so I've seen every barrette, bally and hairstyle you can imagine that dresses black hair. I have seen various styles of black hair—even the synthetic and Indian hair that tends to cover the black hair of some men and many women. Many women I encounter find the fact that I know about hot oil treatments, various weave installation processes, press-n-curls and other hairstyles quite humorous.

My mother has done my hair for as long as I've had any. There were not many times that my own hair was not either braided or twisted. I have not had many haircuts in my lifetime because my mother and I had a deal. If my grades dropped, then I had to cut my hair off. Apparently, I have done pretty well since I have only had *two* haircuts since that deal eight years ago. For my fifth-grade graduation, she braided the numbers 2003 into my hair. For my older cousin's high school graduation, she braided the numbers 2008 in the back and the letters J-A-S-O-N in the front. From those moments, and aside from being a momma's boy, I knew that my mom was the only person who will do my hair.

Now I have medium-length brown dreadlocks with auburn-colored tips that are home to shells from the sea and saturated with culture from Jamaica and Belize. There are two reasons I chose to go dread. The first was because once my mom's clientele started to build, the times when I was able to get my hair done began to shrink. The second reason was because I was going off to college, and I did not trust anyone to do my hair besides me or my mother. Since I was going to college five hours away, I felt dreadlocks would be the easiest for me to maintain. I am able to place them in a ponytail and get them braided or even plaited. I plan to keep my dreadlocks until the end of time. My only regret is not getting my dreadlocks while my hair was short, because we used a tool to install the dreads, and it took forever to complete them.

> One time I met the mother of a young woman who directly told me, "If you want to make it in life you are going to have to cut your hair—look at Obama."

My hairstyle is beneficial in different parts of my life but in others, it may cause problems. When it comes to things like dating, I feel that my hair is a plus. I rarely get any negative feedback—but one time I met the mother of a young woman who directly told me, "If you want to make it in life you are going to have to cut your hair—look at Obama." Usually the typical assumption is to ask if I am Jamaican, which is not a problem because I am a descendent of Jamaican culture (Rastafarian principles). Having dreadlocks is very convenient for me; I can retighten my own hair and occasionally line it up as well. Therefore, in the event that I have a date, I do not have any major panic attacks about my hair—I have my childhood days in the hair salon to thank for that! Even the fact that I know so much about hair makes room for conversation. On another note, most young women I run across *do* typically look for guys with short haircuts. (Usually their types are the ones with fades or an even-all-over style.) This is not to say that this causes any major problems for social life because my personality is one that attracts many people.

Although I was exposed to various styles of hair as young man, it is hard now to be both creative with my hairstyles as well as "professional." There is an invisible line in life that says those two cannot co-exist. I want to be a motivational speaker and an author—but unfortunately, not many people think that braids and dreadlocks are hairstyles for male professionals. Potentially, this may cause controversy for me if I happen to be on television or in a professional atmosphere. Nevertheless, with people like Jeff Johnson and Dr. Cornel West making a positive name for the natural style, I am sure to have a chance. I believe that it is not the hair that makes a person professional but it is their character. I, of course, do take into consideration that hair must be presentable on the business scene; however, there should not be a generic format for what "professional" hairstyles are. With my dreadlocks, I can further pave the way for men with hair to be respected in the business world.

> It is hard now to be both creative with my hairstyles as well as "professional." There is an invisible line in life that says those two cannot co-exist.

With regard to my personal feelings about my hair, I have a deep emotional attachment to it. I feel that my dreads represent the journey of my life. From my days sitting at the salon and now at Arizona State University, my hair has always been a big part of my life. No one can tell me that black hair is not good hair. If my hair is healthy and strong, then it is good, regardless of how silky it may not be. My hair has opened doors for me and has also made some doors a lot harder for me to enter. My hair is a part of who I am; when people describe me, I guarantee that my hair will be included in the description. No matter what challenges occur, my hair will always be a part of me. My black (hair) is beautiful.

> My hair has opened doors for me and has also made some doors a lot harder for me to enter.

Learning to Love
the Curls
Bahareh Abhari

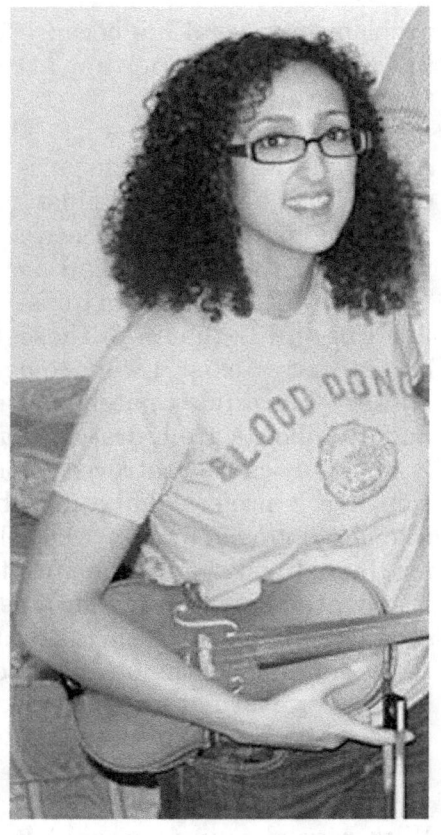

EVEN as I first ventured into the world as a child, I felt that I had committed something intolerable. When I was seven years old, I showed a photograph of me and my Asian-American friend to someone at school. "That's me," I said, pointing to my Asian friend in the picture.

Then, when I was ten years old and playing on the school playground with some younger friends, one of the first graders said to me, "Wow, look at your hair, and look at my hair!" She was only six, but she didn't need to say anything more. I knew what she was telling me: I was something unacceptable.

Sixth grade was around the time in my life when I began to really consider the way I looked. Getting ready for my first party, I turned to my mother for a little assistance.

"What should I do with my hair?" I asked. "I want to wear it down, but it'll get so big when it dries!"

She insisted that it would look beautiful if I wore it down, but I didn't believe her. How could she say that with her perfectly straight relaxed hair?

"Faghad ye khorde tekonesh bede, melse doggy," she replied to me in Persian.

Was she serious? Shake my hair like a wet dog? Even after her high-tech procedures, I decided my hair was WAY too big, as usual, and I needed to put it back up again. My hair needed to be put away.

At age twelve, I began pleading with my mother to relax my hair too. She finally gave in, and I was ecstatic! I could finally look like my mother and my girlfriends at school. Best of all, for all of the girls, the boys, the kids and the adults, I would finally look acceptable. And I would be *pretty*. My hair remained in this form, damaged as it was, well into high school.

During this time, I first encountered a friend who had hair similar to mine. Together, we attempted to battle my hair into submission time and time again. Sometimes we had to just give up. While practicing our swingy-hair dance moves for the high school dance team, my friend would laugh and say, "Bahareh, don't even try to do that, you don't have white people hair!" Again the concept of "acceptable" came to mind. It was made clear to me that even pretending to have straight hair was not good enough.

A wonderful breakthrough (or setback) in college changed everything: THERMAL STRAIGHTENING. Yes, I could straighten my hair without the "chemical" look. Most of my undergraduate college years were spent with this straightened hair texture. But I was no longer happy with this brittle, forever-shoulder-length hair. A change had to be made. I had had chemically straightened hair for most of my adolescence and adult life. What was I, underneath all of that?

Thus began the growing-out phase. For six months, I lived in the limbo of this ugly transition phase. I had no idea what to do. I had never had to deal with any kind of transitioning of curls or anything of that nature until that point. Finally, it just

> I had had chemically straightened hair for most of my adolescence and adult life. What was I, underneath all of that?

became so hideous that the only option I had left was to cut off the straight ends. Later I came to find that this act was known as the Big Chop. To know that other women have experienced such an event in their lives, an event so important that it has its own name, led to a lovely resonating feeling.

That pivotal event marked the beginning of the three-year period in which I have been expressing myself in a new, unapologetic way. At first, it was such a rebellious feeling, but now doing this has emboldened me to ask, *Why was this hair not acceptable? Who made it so?*

> I have been expressing myself in a new, unapologetic way.

To celebrate my newfound self-acceptance, I participated in a photo project about personal insecurities called the What I Be project. I proudly exclaimed in the photo, "I am not my hair," only to find that it has been said before—not only by the famed, but by unheard men and women of color.

A Journey Through the Times
Charlotte Bruce

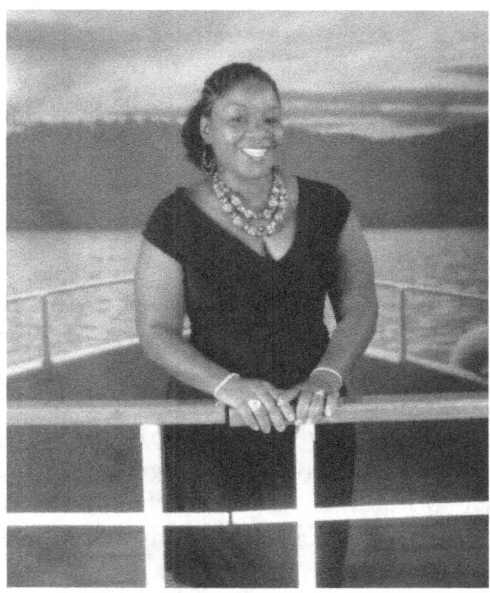

I GREW up in a household with four other sisters. I was my Mom's eighth child and her fifth daughter. The kitchen always smelled of hair grease and burning hair.

On a few occasions I was given a kiddie perm. This did not last long for whatever reason, and it was back to the hot comb, which encouraged my belief that silky curly or silky straight hair was totally acceptable and that my natural kinky hair was beyond unacceptable. My hair was straightened until the mighty Jheri Curl became popular in our house around 1984. This was the last time I saw MY hair before beginning my natural journey in 2007 and going cold turkey from perms, texturizers and heat in 2009.

I LOVED the Jheri Curl. I went from the beginning short curl and ended up with a bob cut (long on one side/short on the other) and a tail shaped into a V in the back. THAT was cool— or so I thought. I had numerous hairdressers, licensed and not licensed, who did my "retouches" as we called them—a four-to-six-hour transformation. Teri was a popular beautician who warned you that she "drenched" her clients. Teri had her Jheri Curl clients wear a poncho over

> Teri was a popular beautician who warned you that she "drenched" her clients. Teri had her Jheri Curl clients wear a poncho over their clothes—and she did indeed drench her clients.

their clothes—and she did indeed drench her clients. I ignorant-
ly thought that the tips of my hair turning blond was cool, too. I
was too young and self-absorbed in my looks to think about what
in the world kind of chemicals would do that?!!

I sported "The Curl" for about three years, but by the time I hit
high school it was time for a change. I transitioned to the almighty
perm! I recall going to the salon and advising my beautician of
my wishes to transition to an official perm for high school, and
she obliged. By this time, my curl was pretty long, and my brain
was washed with the idea that long hair was a necessity. I allowed my new growth to come in for a longer period, not knowing if she would have to cut it all off. She actually put the perm
right in and my hair was gorgeous. Still long on one side/short on
the other and a good length in the back. Thinking back on this,
it was a miracle that my hair did not immediately fall out.

But it did eventually fall out.

The long side of my bobbed cut was the first to go. I was able to
hide the bald spot for a while with the layer above it. But right
around the time that Anita Baker was in her prime, I knew that
there was only one thing to do. Get an Anita Baker haircut. Short
hair now acceptable! But, unfortunately, the balding I had required that my hair be cut much shorter. With the short cut, it
HAD to be layered perfectly and bone straight. If a twinge of it
curled up, I permed it.

After graduation, I did some of everything with my hair, including scrunches, weave ponytails, braids, pincurls, French rolls,
and various colors and perm brands . . . you name it. I eventually
grew weary of the hair breakage and the perms that seemed to
not last, and I started my transition to natural hair. I started
out by using texturizers and kiddie perms every two months and
then every four months. I started wearing half-wigs as I knew
nothing about natural hair. In the summer of 2009 came the Big
Chop, and I let go of the texturizers completely. I did this myself.
It wasn't too hard because I clipped the permed hair out slowly
from time to time. By the time I cut out the remainder, my un-
permed hair was longer than the permed portion.

People's reactions were mixed. My husband was simply happy that I was not paying someone megabucks to do my hair. One of my sisters was very happy as she already had natural hair. *Good hair* . . . as they call it. My mom has transitioned too, so she likes it. Another sister was still going through the transitioning process and was happy to see what she was in for as her hair was just as coarse as my own. We both agree that we have the coarsest hair on earth. KNOTTY! But I've learned to love mine. At thirty-nine, I have finally accepted my natural hair. I am now wearing my natural out daily. No more lacefront weaves!

> At thirty-nine, I have finally accepted my natural hair. I am now wearing my natural out daily. No more lacefront weaves!

Caring for my natural hair was and still is somewhat challenging. After years of chemicals, it is hard to work with what is natural. That even sounds backwards, but it is what it is. Many licensed beauticians don't want to treat or style natural hair. The ones who will only want to straighten it with a hot comb or hand dryer. I've heard from one that it is just not profitable.

> I have accepted that my hair is beautiful, thick, black, dependable, ever-growing, stable, stylish; it does not care what people think and owes no explanation for its current or future state.

I have accepted that my hair is beautiful, thick, black, dependable, ever-growing, stable, stylish; it does not care what people think and owes no explanation for its current or future state. That's me! My hair is GOOD. In fact it is "gooder" than good!

Invisible Beauty
Amber May

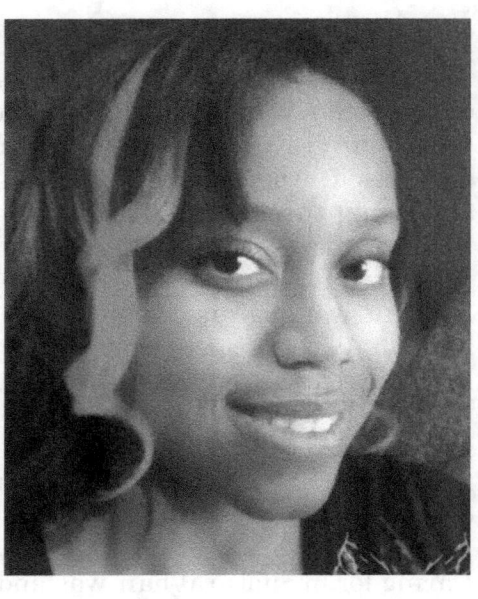

THE most common stereotypical traits for African-American women are their luscious backsides, their loud mouths and their fabulously styled hair. I, sadly, lack all three of these traits. My backside is flatter than a chalkboard, my voice is quieter than a mouse during a church service, and my hair is always either in a short ponytail or hanging loose on my shoulders, nothing fancy. In school, I felt as if I had been left out from something really important—I just couldn't figure out what it was. I was just "that black girl without a name."

I did, every so often, look at the other girls' bodies and wish that my body was just like theirs. What really caught my attention were their stunning hairstyles. Their hair flowed with endless curls and twists, some jet-black and others in a variety of colors. Some of these girls spent over sixty dollars *per week* getting their hair done! I would remember how bland and monotonous my hair looked, and this was my motivation to change something. I realized that I was just another piece of hay in the haystack. No more would I be that invisible person who occupied a seat in class. With this thought floating through my mind, I went home that evening and plotted my transformation. When the plan was complete, I asked my mom for advice about it. She just shook her head and said, "Amber, you're a senior in high school now. You can do whatever you want to your hair."

Once I received the okay, I excitedly drove to the hair shop to pick up some supplies and then to the beauty salon to meet with my usual beautician. She greeted me and asked, "Are we doing the usual today?" I shook my head and explained my idea. She just gave me a look and asked if I had my mom's permission. I nodded and gave her the supplies I'd bought. The process of relaxing, shampooing, trimming, curling and gluing took about three hours. At the end of the procedure, my beautician was shocked at how gorgeous and different I looked. She handed me a mirror and asked how I liked it. I paused for a second and replied, "This . . . is . . . *AWESOME*!" My hair was different from my usual ponytail; it was curled, flatironed and shimmering. However, it wasn't the style that got people's attention, it was the hot pink that was beautifully woven through my hair. Other clients in the salon looked at my hair and instantly loved it; some wanted their own hair in the same fashion. This was only the beginning, though. My real test was how my classmates would react the next day at school.

The hairstyle and color I had was probably common, but just the fact that *I*—the one who usually doesn't care about looks—had this style amazed others at school the next day. As I walked through the halls, people were looking at me for the first time as if I weren't invisible! Being the shy nerd that I was, it made me nervous to have so many students watching me, their eyes piercing my skin. I awkwardly tried to hide my face by staring at the wall as I walked, which was a bad idea because I ended up walking right into one of the cutest boys in our class. I must have apologized a million times to him and gave him a million excuses for my clumsiness! He just smiled, picked up one of the books I'd dropped and glanced at me for a second with his ocean-blue eyes. Thoughts were racing in my mind: *Oh my God! Why's he looking at me? Do I have something in my teeth? Maybe he thinks I look ugly! I should just walk away from him! I'm such a dork!*

> The hairstyle and color I had was probably common, but just the fact that *I*—the one who usually doesn't care about looks—had this style amazed others at school the next day.

I was about to apologize one more time, but he had already started introducing himself and asking what my name was. I nervously told him my name, avoiding eye contact with him. I was still overwhelmed by the fact that I was having an actual conversation with the cutest guy in school. The bell rang for first period to start, so we both said how it was nice meeting each other and walked in different directions. Before I left, however, he turned around and delightfully said, "Oh, by the way, I love that color in your hair. It goes with that sweet smile of yours." The rest of my day consisted of words like *gorgeous, attractive and amazing*— words that I'd never heard anyone besides my family call me.

Surprisingly, at the end of that day—I was downhearted. It reminded me of how much looks played a major role in the development of social reputation. However, it took me until that day when I changed my hair to completely understand that it's not what's on the outside that is important. It is what's on the inside that makes a person an individual and sets them apart from others. God created each and every one of us in his own image, and like snowflakes, all of us are unique and have our own inner beauty. I guess this is why I never wore makeup or spent hours working toward physical beauty and perfection. If I had the choice between having hundreds of fake friends who only like me solely for my looks or staying invisible and having a couple of friends who like me for who I am, I would choose the latter and be happy to call myself "just that black chick."

> God created each and every one of us in his own image, and like snowflakes, all of us are unique and have our own inner beauty.

On Finding My Hair Identity
Darian Washington

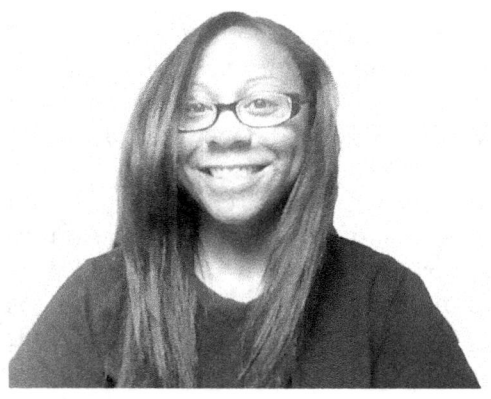

M Y feelings toward my hair are just as indecisive as California weather. Throughout my youth, I was praised for having "good" hair. My mother would brag to her friends about it, my grandmother would call me lucky and my dad would take all the credit. I never knew what it meant, but I took it and ran with it. My friends were jealous. I indulged the attention and thought I was on top of the world. Then, one day in seventh grade, my overdramatized soap-opera life turned upside down.

One of my best friends was experiencing heartbreak. The boy she liked didn't want to sit next to her on the bus because she had *nappy* hair. This was my first encounter with the term nappy. I had never taken the time to think that if I had "good" hair, then "bad" hair existed as well. I saw how something as simple as hair made my friends self-conscious. This is where the internal battle with my hair began. I wanted to be proud of my hair, but I didn't want to make other girls feel bad about their hair. Another rude awakening was soon to come.

> I was praised for having "good" hair. My mother would brag to her friends about it, my grandmother would call me lucky and my dad would take all the credit.

High school was a whole new ball game. Girls had perms! This was another new concept for me. My naturally curly hair was no match for a fresh perm, press and curl. My participation in swim team and water polo never allowed me to straighten my hair. I no longer received the same amount of attention as I did in middle school. For this portion of my life, I pretty much loathed my hair. My self-esteem plummeted. My social interaction decreased as well.

My father noticed how withdrawn I had become and allowed me to get a relaxer. He lectured me about how I should accept my hair as it was and that real beauty was on the inside—but I felt that this was a mandatory speech all parents had to give. I will never forget my mother's reaction. I walked into the house boasting to my friend on the phone, and she sat at the end of the kitchen table glaring at my father with tears in her eyes. I never really knew why she was mad; I was just happy my dad was the one in trouble and not me. Sadly, my relaxer didn't make me any more confident AND it caused most of my hair to break off. Hair that once flowed down my back I now combed out in chunks every day after washing my hair. Needless to say, I was devastated. I had been sure that a relaxer was my path to happiness.

> I had never taken the time to think that if I had "good" hair, then "bad" hair existed as well.

College was the next step, and I was leery of what my sister called "finding your identity." As always, my sister was right. I found my swag in college! Natural again, I tried new hairstyles with my hair: Updos, wash and gos, twist-outs, bantu knots and all the like. I really took the time to find out what I thought looked good. This was the key! It only mattered what I thought. I noticed how more men would approach me when my hair was straightened than when curly. I pondered the reasons why but ultimately gave up. My hair was complicated enough; I couldn't add men to the mix too.

Since then I have dedicated time to learning about keeping my hair healthy. In the present, I work to find the right mixture of products to use that will optimize my curls and protect my hair from the heat when I do decide to straighten it. Although my hair and I have hiccups in our relationship, we have learned to compromise, and it all works out at the end of the day.

Hair Escapades
Dominique Allen

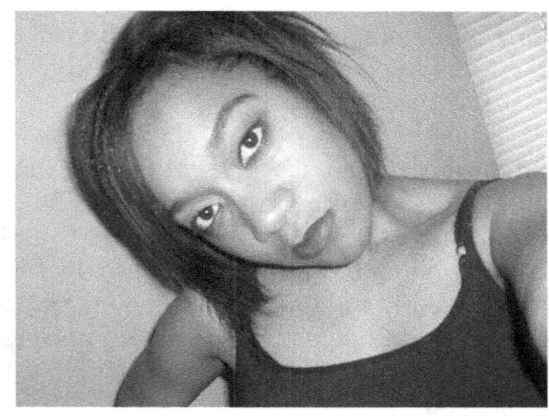

SINCE the beginning of time, women have been told that their hair is their glory, strength and beauty. As a result, women have put a great amount of time into tending to their hair and making sure that it is up to date with the style of the time. Hair is especially important within the African-American community. African-American women put a lot of money into their hair and all that comes along with it. This has been no different for me.

As a child, my hair was natural. When I was a baby, I would wear it in two small Afro ponytails. As my hair grew, I began to wear my hair in little plaits (usually two or three) that were pressed out.

My mom usually did my hair, but as I got older, it became a more painful process. So, at the age of ten, we decided that I should get a texturizer because it would be less stress on both of us. Of course, I was excited that I would finally be getting one. What I did not know, however, was all of the problems that would follow this new and exciting thing. At first, my hair had grown down to the midpoint of my back—but a best friend of my mother's started doing my hair and accidentally burned it out. I kissed my good long hair goodbye, and the process of my hair recovery began.

Over time, my hair became overprocessed and really thin from the texturizers, so my mom and I decided that I should go a while without getting any type of chemical put in my hair to let my hair rest. I really wanted to go natural because I was tired of the chemicals, and I wanted to wear my real and unprocessed hair. I no longer believed in getting perms or trying to look a certain way. If people did not like my natural hair, they would just have to deal with it.

So, I went along with this natural hair mentality until one summer, while staying with my aunt, my hair began to annoy me so much that I let her give me a perm. She thought she knew what she was doing but pulled it all the way through to the ends of my hair, causing my hair to become overprocessed yet again. After that, I again decided that I would not put any kind of chemical in my hair at all. Instead of cutting out the perm, I just let my hair grow out.

During this time, the hair that began to grow in was thick (because it was natural). Since I did not want to put a chemical on it, my mom decided to try to press it out with a hot comb. She placed the hot comb on top of our kitchen stove and then proceeded to press my hair. As soon as the comb touched my hair, we heard my hair begin to sizzle. She pulled away the hot comb as quickly as possible, but it had already burned some of my hair out and the color was now gone too. I remember feeling so down and not wanting to do anything but lie in my bed and cry the whole day. Instead of going to school that day, we went to the grocery store and bought brown hair dye. It ended up looking red, but I dealt with it because at least it looked better than it had previously.

> I would love to go natural again one day, but I know that I have to be prepared for it.

After that incident, I went a while without putting a texturizer in my hair—but my boyfriend wanted me to go to prom with him, so I got another texturizer so that I would look semipresentable at the prom. I had a new thick and beautiful head of hair, and I was really happy with how it turned out. It has been growing ever since that day. I would love to go natural again one day, but I know that I have to be prepared for it.

My hair has had a part to play in who I am today because my "hair escapades" have shown me that no matter what is on my head, I am still the same person. We have to think for ourselves and decide whether we want to be remembered for our hair—or for the impact we left on the world and those around us. No matter what people say, we are beautiful, regardless of what kind of hair we have, whether it is fake or real, long or short, thick or thin, nappy or fine. What matters most is what is on the inside, not on the outside.

> We have to think for ourselves and decide whether we want to be remembered for our hair—or for the impact we left on the world and those around us.

Learning to Love "Bad Hair"
Melissa Glenn Tran-Coley

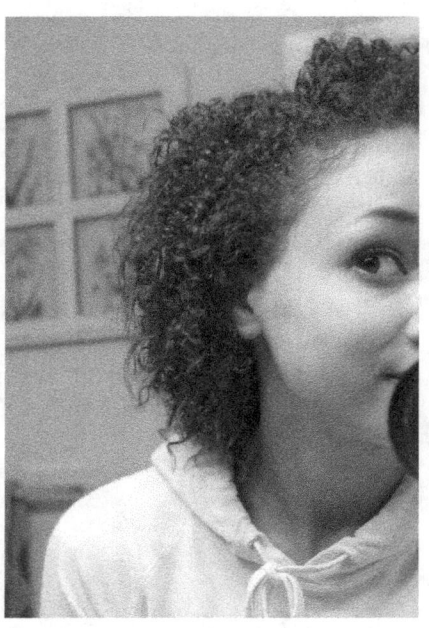

My road to hair acceptance has been anything but a smooth one. With being biracial, there's always that misconception that you have the perfect loose-ringletted, long, curly hair, which was not the case at all for me. I actually used to refer to my hair as the "bad biracial hair"—very tightly curled and slow-to-grow hair.

Needless to say, I spent most of my childhood with my hair tied up in either pigtails or braids. I would go to sleep with hopes of waking up with long, straight, beautiful "good hair" like all my little (white) friends. I remember on the rare occasion when I did wear my hair down, I would be the butt of all the kids' jokes. They'd ask me what the thing or monster on my head was or ask why I didn't comb my hair. Looking back now, I wish I could have been more confident with myself. I wish I would have just brushed their hurtful comments off and not given them much thought. Little did those kids know how much their jokes would affect my self-esteem in the years to come.

> With being biracial, there's always that misconception that you have the perfect loose-ringletted, long, curly hair.

Middle school was when I discovered the art of flatironing and being able to transform my curly hair into what I thought was silky, shiny, beautiful, perfect hair like the hair of my friends. I looked past the fact that I had to wake up at 5 A.M. to begin the hour-and-a-half-long process—and the fact that I had to keep my eyes glued on The Weather Channel and pray for no chance of rain—and the fact that by the end of the day, all my efforts couldn't keep my hair from frizzing up. I looked past all this because for the first time, I felt pretty and like I fit in. I became so obsessed with straightening my hair and never letting *anyone* see my curly mess in its natural form that many of my new friends didn't even know my hair wasn't naturally straight. They just assumed it was. I remember lying in P.E. class and saying that I couldn't swim just so I didn't have to get my hair wet and expose my curly secret. I failed P.E., but I was just happy my hair was safe.

> They'd ask me what the thing or monster on my head was or ask why I didn't comb my hair.

> I looked past the fact that I had to wake up at 5 A.M. to begin the hour-and-a-half-long process—and the fact that I had to keep my eyes glued on The Weather Channel and pray for no chance of rain—and the fact that by the end of the day, all my efforts couldn't keep my hair from frizzing up.

As silly as it sounds now, my hair was a major source of pain and frustration throughout the years. I don't know when it clicked for me, but I now understand that instead of fighting against my curls, I need to work with them. Instead of treating my hair like what I wished it was, I accepted it for what it is. It's been a long time coming, but I can finally say I love my hair. Even as high-maintenance, difficult and time-consuming as it can be, I love every curl.

Defining My Own Beauty
Shakeda Muldrow

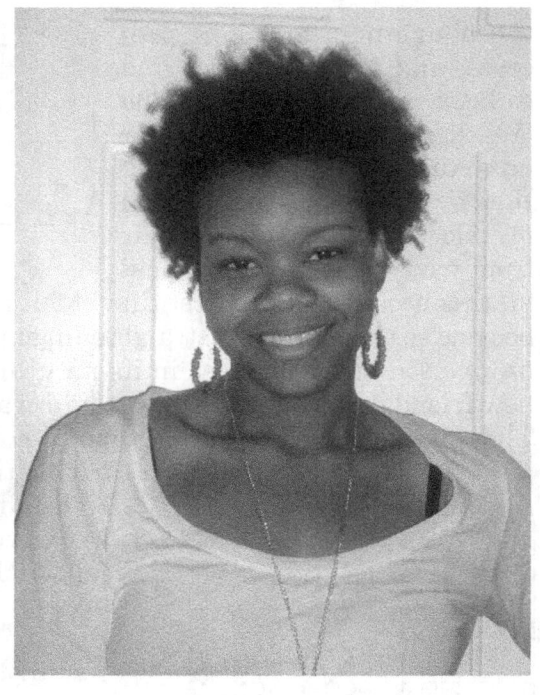

GOING from relaxed to natural hair was one of the best decisions I could ever have made. It opened my eyes to see that there is more than one look of beauty for myself and other African-American females.

I remember when I first considered going natural. I was a sophomore in college. My African-American history professor had dreads and was sharing her story of why she went natural. While she was speaking, I started picturing myself with an Afro or with dreads and immediately killed the idea from going any further. I thought the usual: My face is too fat, my head is too big—but in actuality the issue was that I could not see the beauty of natural hair because I had never been exposed to anything else other than relaxers from childhood.

As a child, and up into my late adolescent years, I struggled with having my own definition and perception of beauty. I am confident that many African-American females have had similar experiences. With sitcoms, commercials and magazines highlighting the features of the majority population, it is extremely hard for African-American females to perceive their own beauty. I remember being in school and wishing my hair was long and bouncy like the hair of my white and biracial classmates. I thought I would be prettier with hair like theirs. For years, I walked around believing I was less beautiful because I had equated beauty with their hair and was convinced there was nothing more accentu-ating to a female than the length and flow of her hair.

When I finally decided to go natural, I was a senior in college and chose to do so believing that it would be healthier for my hair. The process of going natural was difficult, but even more challenging was wearing my hair in a style other than a wrap or roller set. Instead of doing the Big Chop, I chose to grow my relaxer out. The first phase was easy main-tenance because I had a sewn-in weave, but once the weave was out, the challenge began. For the next several months I kept my hair pressed while my beautician trimmed my ends, gradually cutting the perm away.

> I started picturing myself with an Afro or with dreads and immediately killed the idea from going any further.

Reuniting with a hot comb was challenging. Even more challeng-ing was that I had to learn how to keep my hair from swelling in the hot and humid heat of the South. There were several oc-casions when I thought I should just get a relaxer because of all the maintenance my hair required during its transition. I per-severed. I kept my hair pressed throughout the entire summer, and once it began to cool down, I decided to get braids until the rest of my relaxer grew out. Still longing for long, bouncy hair, I continued getting my hair straightened once it was completely natural. Although my hair had made the transition, my mind had not. I still equated beauty with lengthy, flowing hair and was concerned about how others would view me—and more im-portantly, how I would view myself.

I knew very little about the upkeep of natural hair. One of my girlfriends who had been natural for five years wore her hair in an Afro, braids, twists and other creative styles. I wondered how an Afro would look on me, and although I was not completely comfortable with the idea, I knew that I had worked too hard growing my relaxer out not to try something new. Since I was too nervous about wearing my hair in an actual Afro, I had it styled with straw curls to get an idea of how it might look. At first I did not like it. I was not used to seeing my hair so short and tight—but I had paid for it, so I kept the hairstyle. I became fond of it as time went by. Feeling better about my hair, I decided to take a big step and wear it out in an Afro using just shea butter and oil. For the first time I actually saw my natural curl pattern, and I was amazed at the textures and pattern of my hair. My mind started to shift, and I began to develop an appreciation of and higher level of confidence about myself and my hair. The thought of having long and bouncy hair was becoming less of a concern. I was starting to define and perceive my own beauty.

Even though I was happy about my hair and enjoying the experience of discovering my own beauty, some people did not respond well to my new look. The first time I came home with my hair in an Afro, my father looked at me and asked in a perplexed voice, "Are you thinking about Africa?" I laughed at his comment and explained to him that my hair was natural. He told me he did not like it, and that I needed to change it back. My sister told me it would look better if it

> Although my hair had made the transition, my mind had not.

were longer. Some men even told me that I looked better when my hair was straightened and that they were not attracted to women with natural hair. I tried my best to explain how going natural is a liberating experience for black females, but they did not seem to understand. None of these comments could compare with how great I felt about myself and how empowering and encouraging it is to see other African-American females embrace their natural hair.

I strongly advise any female that is curious about going natural to try it. I am convinced that I will never go back to a relaxer. I am more confident than I have ever been, and I love the versatility of my hair. With a relaxer I was limited to certain styles, but now I can wear it braided, twisted or straightened, taking my hair on any adventure I feel like having. Going natural has been a very liberating experience for me, and I am glad this fad is sweeping the nation of African-American females so that they too can discover their own beauty.

Loving the Skin I'm In
Ayres Cook

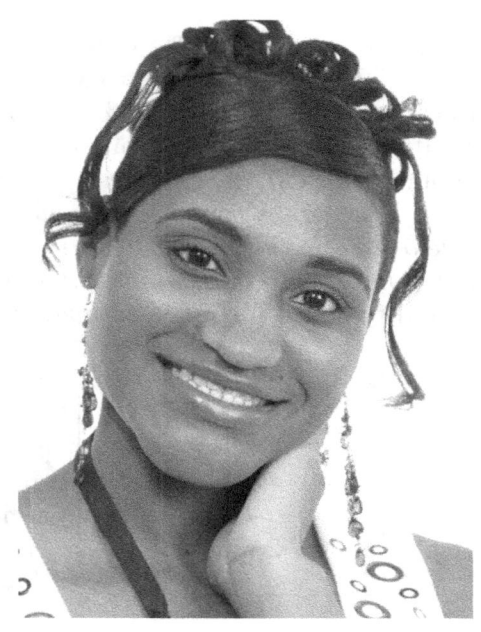

LIFE is about choices, and you can choose to be happy with who you were created to be or choose to make yourself into something that you were not born to be. I choose to embrace my authentic self, my distinguished chin, the remarkable beauty mark on my face, my defined curves, my one-in-a-million smile and, of course, my flawless, healthy hair. I love my hair! My hair is one of the best things about me. My hair is very manageable, healthy and easy to style. It's me, and I love it. I am not a vain person; I was just raised to take pride in my overall being.

At the age of five I had my first relaxer. Since I was so young, I did not know what a relaxer was. I just thought that it was going to make my hair pretty. When I told my mother that I had had a relaxer, her exact words were, "Ayres, what are you talking about, and what was your grandmother thinking?"

Growing up, I used to be very shy and have low self-esteem because I didn't look like the blond models on television. It is a fact that we live in a society that judges people by their physical appearances before really getting to know you. As an African-American woman, society already had two strikes against me: the color of my skin and my gender. However, a major event in my life would make me appreciate who I was and my overall health.

In the summer of 2007, a very freaky accident made me learn to appreciate my life and not to worry so much about what I had or didn't have. The summer before my freshman year of high school, I suffered a third-degree burn on my forehead from a candle. I freaked out. *Oh, my goodness, I thought to myself. My life is ruined. How can I start my freshman year of high school looking like a freak? No one will want to be my friend or hang out with me. I am so ugly—I wish I could hide forever!* But my mother had a reality check for me. She made me watch a "Dateline NBC" T.V. episode in which a woman, a victim of a drunk-driving accident, was burned on over 90 percent of her body. Pretty pictures of this woman before her accident flashed across the television screen. Burned today, all that that lady wanted was to be seen as a human being and not as a monster. While watching that show, my mother said to me, "Ayres, if you become consumed with how you look on the outside, you will become ugly on the inside, and you will be alone in this world." After that, I began to thank God that my own burn was only temporary, not permanent. Although my hair already had had a huge impact on my self-esteem, this showed me that without my hair, I still mattered in life. My hair doesn't define me—it's just an extension of who I am. It's not the beginning, middle or end of me. I am loved and adored by many—not because of my hair, but because of my personality.

> Although my hair already had had a huge impact on my self-esteem, this showed me that without my hair, I still mattered in life.

It has taken me a long time to really be happy in the skin I'm in—but I will embrace who I am because nobody else will ever be able to say, "I am Ayres Marcel Eubanks Cook."

The Love-Hate Struggle
Brittany Biggett

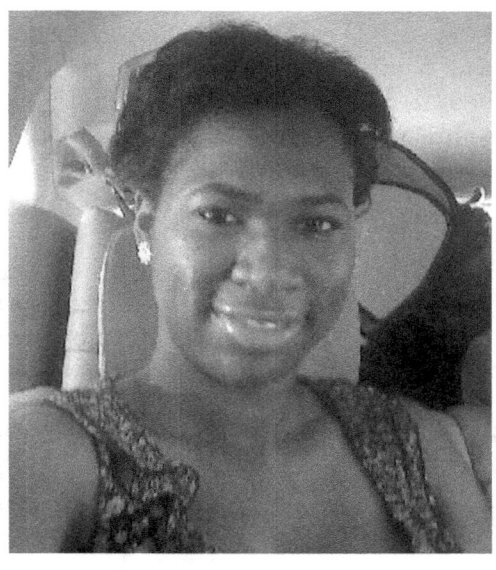

"There are times when I flick through magazines . . . and think I'm in danger of becoming a prisoner of my own hair."
—Brian May

Reading this quote makes me think back through my childhood and about how true it is. I've had a very privileged life, and I am proud of where I came from—but I can say that I have had struggles with myself along the way.

As an African-American female, I was raised in upper-middle-class neighborhoods and schools, so I was surrounded by a majority of Caucasians growing up. My definition of beauty became the girls I saw around me with long, flowing locks and seemingly easy-to-manage hair. I, on the other hand, felt inferior with my naturally wavy hair and on account of not being able to do with my hair what I saw them do. Even though my mother was an example of African-American beauty in my life, her hair texture was more Caucasian, so I felt as though she really couldn't feel my struggle about my hair. As a young girl growing up, I felt inferior and ugly because the boys would talk to the girls with the long, flowing hair. I would just stand there with my braids thinking, *I wish I had her hair. He might talk to me if I had her hair.*

I remember one day at eight years old going to my mother, feeling so insecure and ashamed of my hair, and telling her that I wanted to be white and have long, flowing hair like the girls at school. I will always remember the hurt look my words brought to my mother's eyes. She felt as though she wasn't doing her part in raising a strong African-American female. She told me that I was beautiful, and that my hair and skin made me unique and beautiful. Then one day my mother put a relaxer in my hair—and I went to school the next day and got a different reaction. I felt like I finally belonged with my relaxed hair, and my confidence increased.

As I grew up and exposed myself to other African-Americans with different hair textures, colors and styles, I saw that relaxed was not the only way to be seen as beautiful. I really experienced this when I came to Florida A&M University. Being at a historically black university really made me see the different styles of our hair. I also learned how to manage my hair

> I know that my hair is beautiful and that *I* make my hair.

to keep it looking and feeling healthy. I don't know what the future holds for my hair—whether I'll go natural, keep it short or get a weave—but I know that my hair is beautiful and that I make my hair.

On a Different Kind of Hair Resentment
Jace Ross

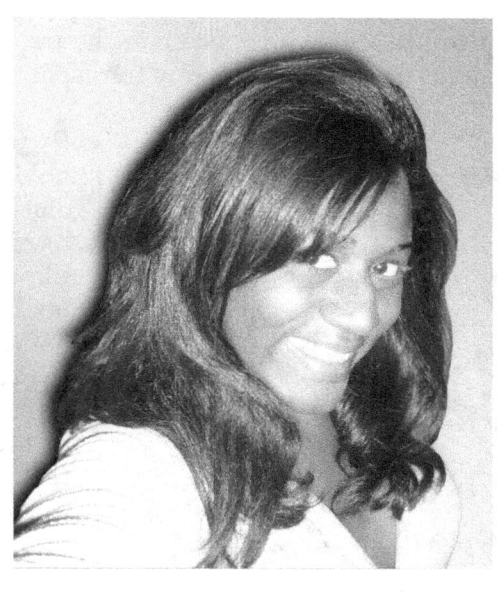

I F it's okay with you, I'd like to start this essay off with a confession. I know we have never met, but I feel obligated to inform you that my hair and I have not always been the best of friends. I will even admit that I used to resent my hair. In fact, I confess that the neglect in our relationship was primarily on my part. Metaphorically, I guess I can say that my hair and I have had a long, coarse, twisted, mangled, tough and, at times, tangled relationship. Let me explain.

I have been blessed with a full head of long hair. My mother, both grandmothers and both great-grandmothers all have similar hair. And yes, it's all ours. To this day I have never used a perm or any other type of texturizing chemical on my hair. I never felt that I was different from any other African-American girl until about the age of five. I was often asked, "Is that all your hair?" or, worse, "Is that really your hair?" The second part of this question was usually, "Are you ALL black?" I was confused by these questions but always answered yes to both as it is the truth. What usually followed my answers was a compliment *of sorts* about how pretty my hair was. Thirteen years later, I am still being asked the same questions. For more than a decade, my hair caused me anxiety and insecurity and made me question my own appearance and beauty. Generally speaking, people would often tell me that my hair was pretty, but never once did they say that I was pretty. They never complimented me on my grades or G.P.A. I rarely heard that I was a fast sprinter or how nice the outfit that I'd spent hours sewing was. It was always about my hair—so I grew to resent it.

> People would often tell me that my hair was pretty, but never once did they say that I was pretty. They never complimented me on my grades or G.P.A. I rarely heard that I was a fast sprinter or how nice the outfit that I'd spent hours sewing was. It was always about my hair—so I grew to resent it.

By puberty, I was a sight to behold! Not only was I wearing glasses and braces with massive hardware, but I was also angry. I knew just how to get even with my hair, and at twelve years old I started to comb it myself. Boy, I was surely going to teach my hair a lesson! By eighth-grade graduation, it was a tangled, teased, broken, damaged and uneven mess! In retrospect, I understand now that my hair reflected how I felt on the inside. *I* was on the losing end of this crazy idea because regardless of what I did to my hair—braid it, flatiron it, or wear it wet and wild—the compliments about my hair never stopped. Couldn't they see that it was damaged? Were they so engrossed in its length that they turned a blind eye to the severe split ends? What was wrong with these people? Eventually I dyed my hair and even came close to cutting it all off. I thought that maybe by altering my hair, I would become an "individual," and that my personality would finally speak louder than my hair's length. Naively, I had the notion that I could change people's opinions of me if I changed the way I looked on the outside. The fact is, I needed to feel better about *me* on the inside, regardless of what others saw or didn't see. I needed to change how I felt about myself.

Prior to entering high school, I looked in the mirror and saw a damaged, weak, dehydrated and frayed person—not the strong leader, healer and good friend that I wanted to be. This moment was telling: I saw that my hair was stronger than I was! My hair should have fallen out a long time ago, but it hadn't; it just kept growing, regardless of how badly I treated it. Halfway through my freshman year, I was not only finally learning to respect my hair, but I also learned a lesson or two from it. By the end of freshman year, I realized that my hair had character, and I wanted to be just like it.

I GOT IT! *It is about what is on my head, but it's not limited to only that. It's also about what's inside my head and what's in my heart.* I blazed through high school, lettering in track and cheerleading. I was a student ambassador and a Eucharistic Minister, and I served as teen president of my local Jack and Jill Chapter. I graduated with a 5.0 G.P.A. and got accepted into my first-choice college, The Fashion Institute of Technology in New York City—in the Presidential Honors program to boot! I've kept my G.P.A. in college above 3.0 while taking eighteen to twenty-one credit hours and doing an internship and volunteer work.

> I realized that my hair had character, and I wanted to be just like it.

As I describe to you my hair, I describe to you myself. I know that we have never met, but I feel obligated to inform you that today my hair and I are not only best friends, we are so much more. My hair and I love and respect each other now and share a unified goal to be the BEST US we can be, always. If I ever get in a rut, I quickly snap out of it when I remind myself that the words *coarse, long, curly, straight, thick, tough, tender, resilient, lustrous, polished* and bouncy not only describe my hair, but also the relationship I have with it! And yes, I am BEAMIN'!

Hair in a Melting Pot
De Keveion Glaspie

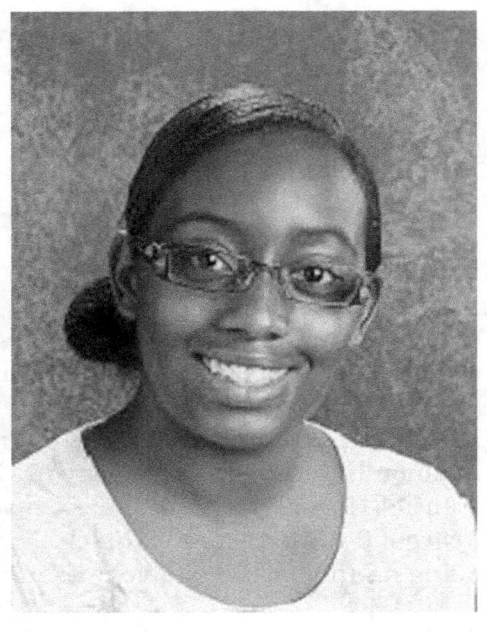

My *hair is different,* I used to say to myself. Growing up, I typically had friends who were not of color— either white or Hispanic. Their hair was always long and soft, while my hair did not grow as much. When they went to the nice salons and got highlights, I was in the kitchen with my mom getting my hair pressed.

Now, if you don't know what this is, let me paint a picture for you. I'm sitting in a chair with my mom over me with a hot comb at the stove and hair grease on the side of my head. So many times I got burnt, and she said it was the grease. Having black hair has always affected me and still does to this day.

I always wanted the long silky hair that I would see on models, but that was something that wasn't so easy to get. Many of the older girls I knew had weaves. That was something I did not like. I didn't even like sitting on a pillow getting braids done with my real hair. Some days, though, when my mom would do my hair, I would look in the mirror and see beauty. The girl I saw in the mirror, though, was not ready for what the people in her future would have to say about her black hair.

As I grew older, I became interested in boys. Living in Colorado, you could say there were many white guys, and you typically get interested in what you are surrounded by. My first boyfriend was white, and he was interested in black girls. The ones after that were also white. None of them had a problem with me or my hair. Some would even say that it was very beautiful.

On the dating subject, nowadays I am interested in Asian guys. When I became interested in Asian guys, some of my black friends would say that they would not like me. I asked why, and they would say because of my dark skin and especially my hair. My friends said Asian guys would say that my hair is too thick and nappy. But my friend, who is Vietnamese, said that what guys think was not based on race or hair, and that every guy in the world has a different opinion.

Another encounter was at a sleepover I was had. A friend who was a foreign exchange student started touching my hair. She asked what it was like having my type of hair. Because it was a new type of hair that she had never seen before, I responded very politely. "I don't know what it is like," I told her. I just take care of it." She smiled and said that it was very nice. I looked at her with confusion. I said, "Thank you," but I was really thinking, *Girl my hair looks like crap. I haven't had a perm on it in weeks.* My friend may not have known this, but her kind words brought such confidence to me. Being a teenager, you tend to go through many phases.

A year ago, when I was sixteen, I wanted to make my hair look like BoA's. She is a Korean pop and hiphop star. To get my hair somewhat like hers, I would have to color it. I begged my mom over and over again to let me go, and I told her I would even pay for it myself. She said that I would have to do it a few weeks after my perm, or my hair would fall out. *Now why is it that every time I want to do something different with my hair, my mom threatens me and says my hair will fall out?* Something I should known then was that my mom was only trying to lookout for me. Otherwise, she would have

> I should have realized years ago that I should be proud of my black hair. It is something that I love and that sets me apart from everyone else.

let me do what I wanted and told me later that it was my fault. My mother is someone I look up to. She may not have long hair, which she knows, but she wears and rocks her hair showing off her beauty in a way that explodes with confidence.

I should have realized years ago that I should be proud of my black hair. It is something that I love and that sets me apart from everyone else. Whether it is long, short, thin or thick, you should be proud of the hair you have. Stand up and show the world what you're working with. Beauty comes in many forms, and mine is only one of them.

Navigating the McKoy Line
Melanie Ray

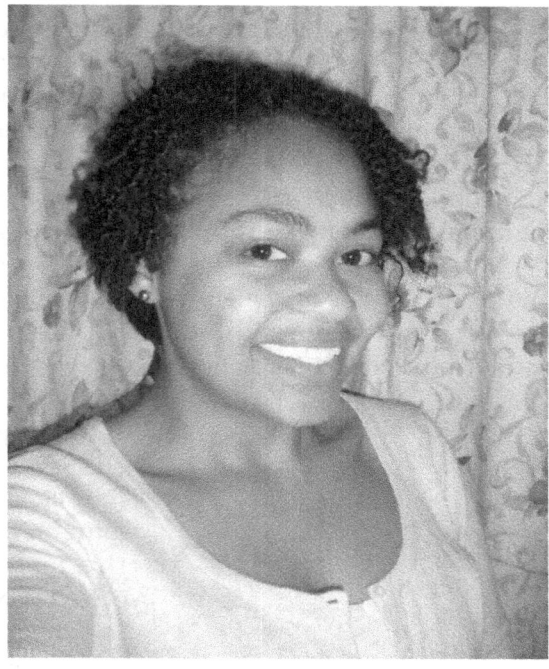

AFROS.
Relaxers.
Weaves.
Locks.
Twists.
Braids.
Tracks.

When it comes to styling hair, black people are certainly the most creative. Our hair, with the help of the different products and procedures available today, can achieve so many unique styles that it may become difficult for others to follow our intentions. In the office, our hair could be straightened and pulled back into a neat bun. For a night on the town, we dramatize our look with a weave that turns heads as soon as we walk into the room. To counter the sweat and humidity of the summer, we can simply braid our hair and keep it oiled. There is no limit to what we can do with our hair.

Of course, it was this versatility that I struggled with throughout my childhood and adolescent years. Like many black mothers in society, my mom refused to let my sister and me relax our hair. She insisted that relaxers led to permanent bald spots and thinned-out hair follicles and would ultimately ruin our thick natural hair. She also warned that if we relaxed our hair, we would fall victim to the "McKoy-line," the receding hairlines that could be seen in each one of my aunts, uncles, cousins and grandparents. This, of course, was something that my sister and I feared!

Now, as a young adult who still embraces her natural hair, I suppose I am grateful that my mom would not allow us to relax our nappy heads. I am still learning of new ways to care for my hair, and I am glad to say that I have not yet inherited the McKoy-line! However, I must admit that despite the advances and changes made in the black hair care industry, it took nearly eighteen years for me to fully accept the versatility of my hair.

In the earlier years of elementary school, things were quite simple in terms of hairstyling. Most young girls styled their hair into braids, cornrows or puffy twists with barrettes. As I recall, everyone wore their hair natural because mothers back then shared the same ideals for black hair care. However, as I entered fourth and fifth grade, I noticed that many of the girls had started to relax their hair. They came to school with their long ponytails and flexi rod curls like they were, as one of my teachers would say, *all that and a bag of chips.* Trying to fit in with the changing style, I asked my mother if I could relax my hair, and she adamantly rejected my request.

> She also warned that if we relaxed our hair, we would fall victim to the "McKoy-line," the receding hairlines that could be seen in each one of my aunts, uncles, cousins and grandparents.

As the girls from elementary school grew older, weaving became a popular trend in black hairstyling. The weaves became more flamboyant throughout my young adolescence, and the extravagance even included experimenting with neon colors! I wondered what my preteen peers were attempting to compensate for with their elaborate designs. One day, in the girls' locker room, I discovered the terrible secret behind every girl's extensions. A girl walked up to me and complimented my two-strand twists. She then asked, "What kind of weave is that?" My reply was, "This is all mine." She could not believe every inch of my long hair was natural, considering that her own hair, which had been relaxed since the fourth grade, was now hidden beneath layers of synthetic hair and was only a couple of inches long! All of that relaxing in elementary school finally began to catch up with these girls, and I could not have been more grateful for my mother's insistence on staying natural. The fact that someone mistook my hair for a weave gave me a small boost of confidence, and I began to think that natural hair was not as bad as society implied it to be.

By the time I entered high school, my pride in natural hair had diminished. *Everyone* decided that relaxing their hair was the only way black women could be socially accepted in America. My friends urged me to "just relax my hair," but I was still somewhat uneasy about such a permanent decision. When I tried out for my high school step team, the pressure only heightened due to the reputation for beauty that the squad had acquired. To the coaches, straight was the only acceptable hairstyle to wear onstage. I felt that this was extremely unfair. Whenever I straightened my hair, the style only lasted a few days—really only a few hours if I performed a series of difficult steps under a hot spotlight.

My main concern, though, was why natural hair could not be accepted as a style of beauty in society. This topic was addressed in the movie *Good Hair* by Chris Rock. After watching it, I started to think about the value placed on relaxed and store-bought hair in the black community. Was I wrong for not relaxing my hair every six weeks? Indeed, my hair would be easier to manage if it were straight, and I would finally fit in with every other young black woman in America. Perhaps I should just cave in. . . .

Since then, I have been in a battle with myself about the status of my hairstyle. In college, I could not dedicate the time that was needed to wash, blow dry and braid my own hair. My hair was too thick, too long and too wild for me to tame it on my own. On the other hand, I did not think a relaxer was the right thing to do for my styling needs. What I needed was a new perspective on natural hair.

That perspective has shaped my opinion of my hair and has just recently become a realization of mine. Natural hair is, in essence, the most versatile look. With my hair in the state it is now, I can virtually style it into any texture and length I desire.

My natural hair has shaped my personality, my lifestyle and my values. I cannot imagine myself without my hair, and although it is in a style that some people still do not deem acceptable, it at least makes me unique.

The Road to Queenhood
Tamaratare Omaya

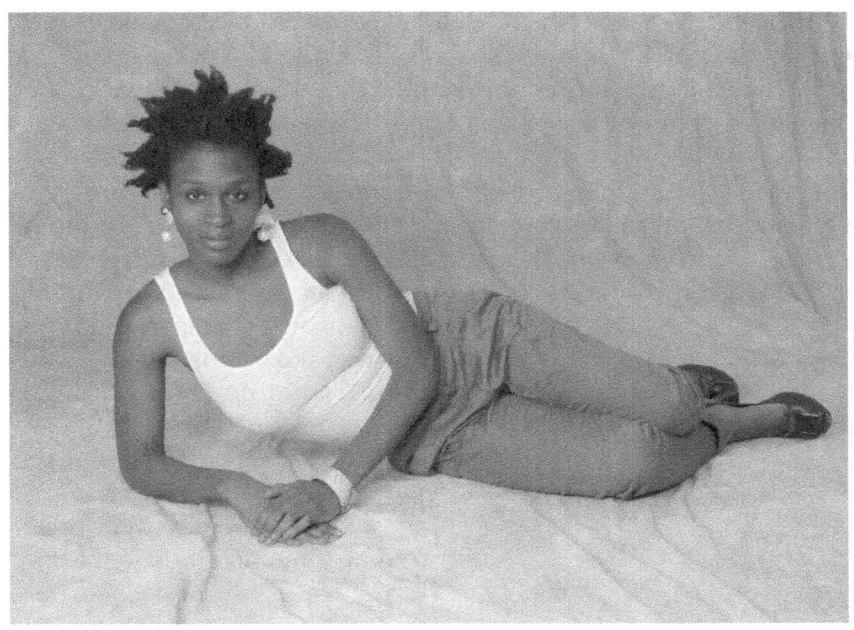

"**O**UCH!!!!"
    "OWWWW, Mom!" I said

"Shut up. I have to finish braiding this tough hair," rebutted my mother.

I got so mad and started to cry silently while my mom slathered hair grease on my scalp. She combed my hair into five sections, braided each section and then wound a native African thread along each braid, banding each braid to the tip of my ends and leaving some thread hanging down. I just sat there looking at the hair grease label and wishing that one day my hair would look as long, silky and soft as the hair of the woman on the hair grease jar.

Growing up, life was really very interesting. I wasn't loved among many for my looks but more for my personality. Actually, many people made fun of me because of the way I looked. I had dark skin, and to add to that, I had short, tightly-coiled, crinkly hair. A comb was hard to get through my thick hair. People called me bald-headed or "beady-bees" and made fun of my skin color. I never saw the beauty in myself. I always waited on others to speak aloud about the beauty in me. I would encourage my friends about their own beauty but refused to see the beauty in myself.

I was only eight years old, when I started to perm my hair myself and get my friends to press and style my hair. My mother was working two jobs and didn't have time to do my hair. I took it into my own hands. I went through phases with kiddie perms, adult perms, regular ponytails, boxbraids, presses and typical children's braided styles. My hair went through severe damage. I had bald spots at the back of my head, thinning in the front, heat damage, perm damage, burns and a lot of hair breakage. My hair looked horrible 90 percent of the time—

> I was only eight years old, when I started to perm my hair myself and get my friends to press and style my hair.

and so I begged teenagers in my neighborhood to do my hair. I actually went around asking people how much they charged and tried to pack bags at the local supermarket to acquire the money. I would go to the local beauty salons, get their cards and find out the prices for different hairstyles. I became obsessed with learning how to style hair.

I was so into hair that I became good at styling it by the fifth grade. I was able to start making money doing other people's hair by the ninth grade. I was fifteen years old, and I got all of my mother's friends' children to come and let me braid their hair. When I learned how to do hair so well, and with my own styles, I got compliments that made me feel shy but amazing at the same time. For once in my life, I was somebody—a beautiful person. I was like a brand-new person, and I didn't want to ever again be judged the way I had been when my hair wasn't done. Around this time in my life, I began to pick my friends based on their looks and how pretty they were. If you were beautiful, with long hair, I would be your friend. I believed that if I were friends with pretty people with long hair, it would take away how bad I felt I looked.

> For once in my life, I was somebody—a beautiful person.

Today, I am a natural Nubian queen who is proud of her natural hue and beauty that's made up of tightly coiled hair and sun-kissed skin. I had to go through life's obstacles in order to be where I am now. I am a confident black woman who is more than just beauty—I have the brains to go with it. My past has made me realize that I must judge people by their character and embrace people's differences in life. I love all people and the uniqueness in society. I am not perfect, but I have wonderful qualities that exemplify a good person. I am caring, spiritual, strong and persistent. I am at the point in my life when I am able to embrace ME wholeheartedly—and naturally!

Loving the
Straight Life
Tatiana Flowers

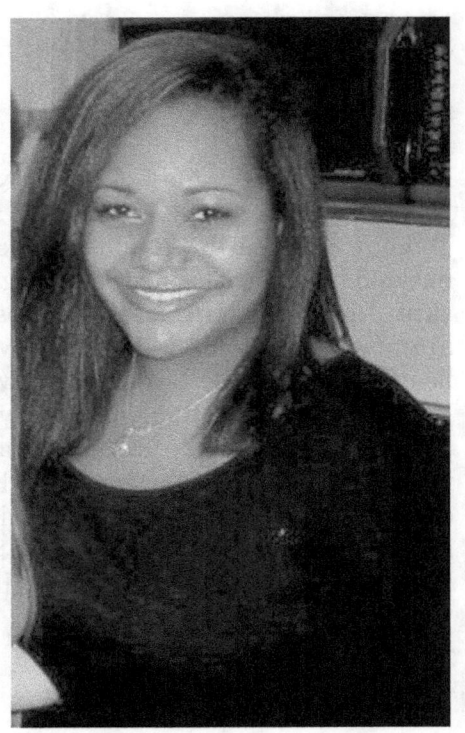

W HEN I was born, my hair was soft and straight as a pin— similar to the hair of someone of Indian descent. As I grew into a toddler, the texture of my hair changed from straight to soft and curly. At that time, it was very manageable; all that my mother had to do was wash and moisturize, and I was ready go. Once I hit the age of three, all havoc broke loose as my hair became impossible to deal with.

My hair's texture was so curly and so thick that each time my mother washed my hair, I would cry and so would she. It took hours at a time to complete my hair routine, and although my mother was never mean to me, she felt that she was when it was time to wash my hair. On those occasions, I despised her as much as she despised washing and blow drying my hair. Her attitude would flare up right before she began my weekly hair regime. The process literally took about three hours from beginning to end. How could that possibly be right? Well, for the first half hour we fought. For the next hour, she washed and untangled my hair. The last hour and a half was dedicated to blow drying, fighting and then styling. Each time my mother said, "Time to wash your hair," my resistance was apparent. Who needed this weekly torture? It was worse than going to nursery school.

> My hair's texture was so curly and so thick that each time my mother washed my hair, I would cry and so would she.

Most mornings when I arrived at school, the students would laugh and say, "You look like an orphan"—not because of my clothing but mainly due to the condition of my hair. I dreaded getting my hair combed, so I devised a plan. My mother worked in Manhattan at the time, and I knew she had to catch a specific train. With precise planning, I created a situation designed to make her late. After missing the train a few times, she started dropping me off at school without combing my hair. This was perfect for me because I did not care what anyone had to say as long as I was not being tortured every single morning.

My mother eventually became hip to my strategy and decided to braid my hair every weekend. This was even more torturous! After washing my hair, she would sit and braid it for hours. The worst part of it all is that my mother is a perfectionist. If one row was a different width from the others, she would take it out and start all over again. At that time, I wished that I was bald because I believed that my hair was the reason for my weekly dysfunctional behavior.

This ordeal lasted about four years in total, and by the time I was seven years old, my mother resorted to perms. She was not experienced in this arena; therefore, she dragged me to her beautician. Almost all of her friends were opposed to the idea of a seven-year old with a perm—but my mother and I were not. It was the best thing she ever did for me, and I am thankful for her early decision. Our relationship grew strong immediately thereafter, and we have become the best of friends. On the opposite side of the spectrum, my father was not a happy camper. From his perspective, perms were made for Caucasian people, not for African-Americans. Time and time again, my father would say, "Be proud of what God blessed you with and stop trying to be white!" He really had no clue as to what my mother and I had dealt with for so many years. In

83

my opinion, his attitude was not about what was right for me but all about his beliefs.

As I progressed through high school, many of my African-American peers made comments about my hair. They would say things like "Do you have a weave?" or "Why does your hair look like the white girls'?" Not understanding why they were asking these questions, I would just continue walking, thinking that maybe they were jealous. My mother has reiterated for many years that I have beautiful, healthy hair and that no matter what anyone says, I should just be proud of who I am. As I reflect back to my younger years, I am happy and thankful for what God has blessed me with. I embrace the fact that there is nothing wrong with relaxing my hair because it has made my life much easier and my hair much more manageable. I love my hair, even when it's wild and crazy!

A Simple,
Feminine Beauty
Kyaunne Richardson

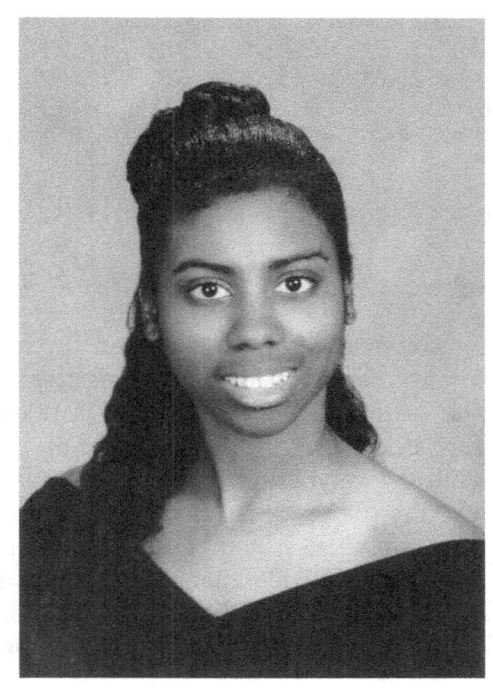

ONE summer day, I was reading a book called *Set-Apart Femininity* by Leslie Ludy. The book addresses the issue of femininity being absent from today's culture. As I read, I came across a chapter called "Sacred Mystique: Femininity That Changes Men into Princes." This chapter caught my attention. As I reflected on this, I realized how much truth was there within the title, how this applied to me as a young woman and how my hair played a key role in affecting the people in my musical environment.

I usually wear a braided style—and when you look at me with my braids, you might assume that I am still in elementary school or about thirteen years old. It's a very simple style. I recall one woman from a local fish market who told me that my hairstyle fits my features; it has become a part of me. I have realized that my style not only fits my features but reflects my personality as kind, sweet, innocent and simple.

It is rare to find young African-American women with long hair that actually belongs to them. I've had people ask if I'm wearing a weave or a wig. I simply replied no and told them that this was my real hair and that, as they can see, there are no chemicals or perms in it. I remember in elementary schoolboys used to pick on me for having braided hair with the bows and trimmings. Other people have told me to wear my hair in a loose style practically

> It is rare to find young African-American women with long hair that actually belongs to them. I've had people ask if I'm wearing a weave or a wig.

every day. There is a particular reason why I do not wear my hair loose and straight every day, and some stories come to mind.

I remember preparing for a concert that was to take place on a Sunday in October 2009. Everyone was trying to figure out what my dress was going to be and the hairstyle I'd wear. I kept it a secret and dropped hints along the way. The day finally arrived, and I came to the theatre in a pink dress and with my hair loose and styled in candy curls. One of my colleagues came up to me and said, "Wow, you look beautiful!" Another time the following year, when I was preparing for my junior recital, I did the same thing with my hair. If you could have seen the looks on their faces—priceless! My colleagues came to me and commented on my singing. "You were wonderful!" they said, and then they commented on my whole style: "You look like a princess!"

Looking back on these memories, I realize it was a challenge for me to understand my feminine uniqueness. I have to laugh but also recognize the reality. While my colleagues continue to discover the secret potential of my hair, I compare their reactions to the experience of a princess being pursued by gallant knight. In the braided hairstyle, I am treated as a regular student; as my braids came loose and my hair is styled to match each musical event, my colleagues' level of protection and respect toward me reach new heights. A wonderful verse comes to mind on this topic: ". . . but that if a woman has long hair, it is her glory? For long hair is given to her as a covering" (1 Corinthians 11:15 [NIV]). Paul talks about how a woman's hair should symbolize her acceptance of the dignity and worth of her womanhood as God created her. A woman looks glorious in her long hair.

My hair is just a factor to heighten my personality since it is a part of me. Through this, I have gained the respect of those around me and shown others the beauty of femininity. In all I do, "I praise you because I am fearfully and wonderfully made; your works are wonderful, I know that full well" (Psalms 139:14 [NIV]).

Soul Searching
Nolita Pore

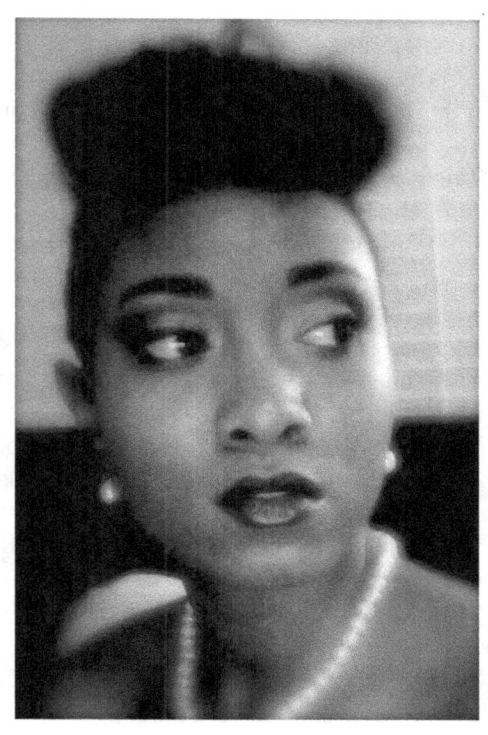

A T a very young age my great-grand-mother said to me, "Nolita, a woman should never cut her hair. It is our crown and glory according to our Lord God." This ideology has been engrained in my subconscious. I have a love-and-hate relationship with my hair at times. There are days when I am in love with my coils and curls, but there are other days when I prefer to have straight hair, so I will flatiron it. I am new to the natural-hair community and still struggling to find the most beneficial hair care routine to help my hair thrive.

When I was nine or ten years old, I begged my mother to relax my hair. I wanted hair just like the young girls on the Just For Me commercials. I thought my curly hair was cute, but it wasn't long enough for me. I would look at my granny, my mom and my cousins, who all had long, thick, pretty hair, and I wanted the same thing for myself. Finally my mother gave in and allowed me to get my hair relaxed. She had a friend from our church do my relaxer. I was really excited and couldn't wait to see the end results. After she applied the relaxer and washed it out, I just knew that my hair would be flowing down my back—but to my surprise, there was no cascading hair. Upset, I turned around in the kitchen chair and asked, "Where is my new hair?"

The church lady responded, "What do you mean?"

I explained to her how I thought that a relaxer was a magical cream that would make hair shoot out of my roots, leaving me with long hair just like the girls from the commercial.

The church lady and my mother both laughed at me. "Little girl, no!" the church lady said." Where did you get that from? A relaxer makes your hair straight, not longer."

I was crushed.

For the next twelve years I continued to relax my hair until I stumbled across a new fascination with my natural texture. During my college study-abroad program in Mexico, I began to do wash and gos. I didn't have access to endless electricity to do roller sets and flatiron my hair constantly, so I had to find a different way of styling my hair. Once I saw the texture of my hair, I became even more curious. When I returned to the States in 2008, I began to transition from relaxed to natural hair.

The journey to become completely natural was a daunting oneand, at times, a test of faith. First, I had an obsession with trying to grow long hair, and I had to do a little soul-searching to overcome this. I was too afraid to cut the remaining relaxed ends off, and I held onto those dead, limp and, quite frankly, raggedy ends until July 3, 2010. The turning point occurred when I had just taken a sewn-in weave out of my hair (another attempt to grow longer hair), only to find that the weave had actually damaged my hair and caused severe breakage.

> As women, we are such complex creatures who are capable of anything that we put our minds to—but at times, we struggle to find peace and serenity in knowing that who we are internally is where our true beauty can be found.

When I saw how much damage had been done to my hair I cried. My attachment to my hair left me feeling unattractive at that moment. After my moment of self-pity, my sorority sister gave me her hairstylist's number, and I called her immediately to schedule a consultation. When I went to the salon for my consultation, the stylist was honest with me and told me that the best thing for me to do was to cut the remaining dead hair off. I was extremely afraid that she would have to cut it so much that I wouldn't recognize myself. Fortunately, the stylist cut my hair into the cutest bob-style haircut, and I absolutely loved it!

The day that stylist cut my hair, I learned something about myself. I learned that my hair didn't make me the beautiful, intelligent, ambitious woman that I am today. As women, we are such complex creatures who are capable of anything that we put our minds to—but at times, we struggle to find peace and serenity in knowing that who we are internally is where our true beauty can be found.

The Quest for
Hassle-Free Hair
Aleah Carr

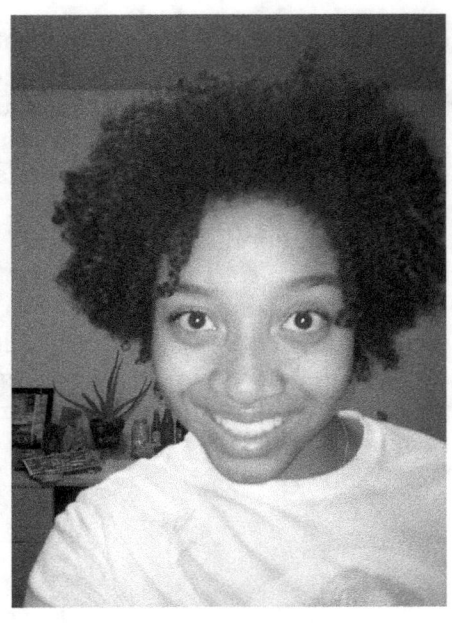

As a child, my hair was always big, curly and tangled! We would spend hours untangling it sometimes, and the only person I really trusted to do it was my mother. Whenever my aunts, cousins or even my dad tried to do my hair, they would yank and pull on it to the point where I would just start crying to make them stop. To solve the problem, I always had my hair braided. I would sit in salon chairs for up to six hours at a time just so we wouldn't have to hassle with it.

That's when my aunt brought up the idea of getting a relaxer so that my hair would be straight and wouldn't get tangled as often. I honestly had no idea what I was doing; I was only eight years old and just wanted pretty, long hair like all my friends. I was tired of being different, and I was always embarrassed because I couldn't wear my hair down like all the other girls. I was so excited to get my hair relaxed. I had never really *felt* pretty but hoped and prayed that by relaxing it I would. I was wrong. Now that I look back, I regret what I did.

Getting my hair relaxed was so much work compared to having it natural. It got harder to straighten with a flatiron, and after a while I just gave up and wore my hair up every day until I decided to cut it into a bob. That's when I started loving my hair again. I still wasn't happy about the fact that it was relaxed, but my new haircut made me feel pretty and unique. I only got it cut like that twice, and then I went back to having it up in a ponytail every day.

The one person who really made me feel beautiful, no matter how my hair looked, was my boyfriend, Eric. He told me I looked beautiful every day, even when I was having a horrible hair day! After a year of dating him, I made the big decision to let my curls grow out and completely cut out my relaxer. I was so nervous that day. When I saw the huge chunks of hair fall to the ground, tears almost came to my eyes. I was so excited to finally have my real hair back, but seeing that much hair float slowly to the ground just broke my heart. I had never felt like that before.

> I was tired of being different, and I was always embarrassed because I couldn't wear my hair down like all the other girls.

About twenty minutes later, I looked in the mirror and saw . . . A LITTLE 'FRO! I felt so cute, I wanted to cry again—but with tears of joy! Even my hairdresser had been nervous to see my reaction, but once I said that I loved my hair, she breathed a sigh of relief and told me that she loved it too. My head felt so light— almost as if I didn't have any hair at all! Eric was also shocked at how much hair had been cut off, but he loved it just as much as I did! I couldn't stop touching it. I had dreamt for so long to see myself with my natural hair.

My curly hair is beautiful, and I love how everyone gives me compliments. I also love when everyone touches and plays with my curls. My hair is unique, like me, and it totally fits my character: I'm wild and crazy, and my hair is definitely wild and crazy!

Becoming One with Nature
Tramaine Paul

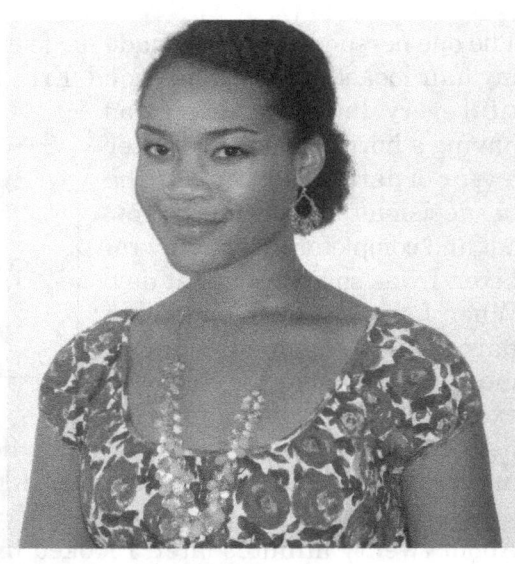

I'VE had a very in-
teresting relation-
ship with my hair.
I've had weaves, po-
nytail extensions and
sew-ins. I've had good
relaxers and bad relax-
ers that left my hair
damaged. All of these
experiences led me to
my current style: nonrelaxed, unstraightened hair.

My hair has affected my self-esteem for as long as I can remember. I did not feel confident about my hair until I was in my mid-
twenties and getting my hair professionally styled every week.
In addition, as an athlete, I never felt feminine enough, and I
usually wore self-procured hair extensions so that I didn't have
to deal with my hair. Now that I am natural, I feel confident *and*
feel that my hair is more consistent and attractive.

Before I went natural, I had lived with chemically processed hair
for twenty-two years. When my sister announced that she was going natural, I laughed. However, after two years, I saw her hair
go from shoulder length to down her back. I stopped laughing and
decided (after understanding that weekly hair appointments were
not feasible for a nonworking graduate student!) that I would go
natural also. It was cheaper. In fact, it was basically free.

I had to change my idea of beauty in others and in myself when
I began to grow my hair out. I had worn my hair straight all
my life, and I did not see many examples of cute girls wearing
their hair curly, unless they had that "mixed" hair or were rocking an exotic or rock look. However, after going through a transition stage while my processed hair grew out, I began to have

problems wearing my straight bob. I transitioned to a strawset and, finally, to wearing my hair natural a year and a half after my last relaxer.

I was astonished by the freedom and the change in my life. I woke up every morning looking forward to exercise. I slept without worrying about how I lay on my hair. I took long showers (twenty minutes!) without a shower cap! I walked in the rain, the wind and the snow (okay, not the snow!). I was one with nature. Even my boyfriend loved the difference. He recalled the times when our schedule and my mood revolved around my hair.

> I was one with nature.

However, I did miss my straight hair. After three months of wearing my hair naturally curly, I decided to straighten it. I was shocked by the fear and trauma that now redescended upon my life. For the next three days, I lived in constant fear of water, wind, sweat, movement and sleep. The only thing that kept me afloat was my vanity. My hair flowed like I was the main girl in a music video. However, I had a secret: I was terrified—terrified that the walk from the car to the office would alter my hair, terrified that the sweat running down my face would cause my hair to expand. Exercise, by the way, was out of the question. When I washed my hair again (I could only take three days of that torture!), I realized that I had always lived like that but just had not realized it. I had always worried about sweating, exercising, sleeping, moving, showering. I realized that something as simple as the style of a person's hair influences a life and could ultimately influence health.

> For the next three days, I lived in constant fear of water, wind, sweat, movement and sleep. The only thing that kept me afloat was my vanity. My hair flowed like I was the main girl in a music video. However, I had a secret: I was terrified.

During my doctoral program, I decided to examine the influence of hair management on exercise frequency among African-

American women as a result of my personal experience with my hair. My assumption, supported by literature, is that for many African-American women, the way we choose to wear our hair influences our activity levels and lifestyles. By focusing on this topic, I bring to the forefront issues that ultimately affect the quality of life of African-American women, in this way hoping to make a difference in my community.

An Eventful Hair Journey

Anastasia Harris

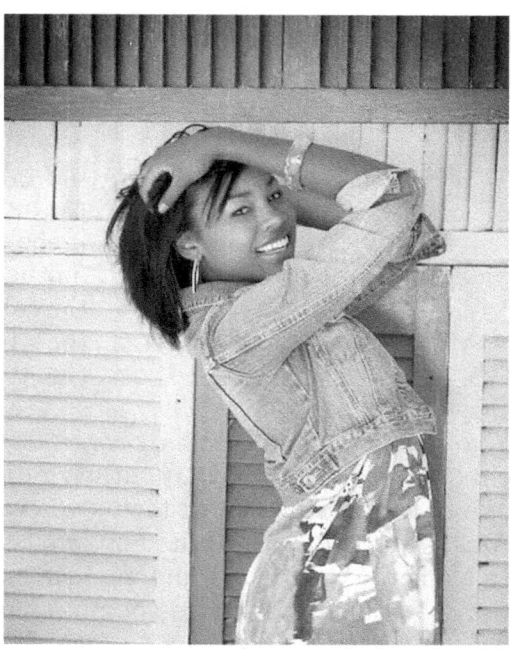

BORN into a society where hair is labeled as either "good" or "bad," a young black girl like me had to find inner confidence—and soon—before I was consumed by the whirlwind of brainwashing about what hair should look like.

On January 20, 1994, when I was born in Howard Medical Hospital in Washington, D.C., I'm told that the nurse muttered, "Wow look at all that hair!" as they gazed at my slick black curls. An Indian boy was born that same night, and the nurses conversed about how similar our hair was. We were almost identical, except for the blue and pink cotton blankets we were wrapped in.

As I smeared white icing all over my face at the age of one, my hair texture was very much the same. My mother kept it separated in ponytails, and my curls burst from those colorful cotton ponytail holders. That was the hairstyle I wore for the next three years, and my mother matched the accessories in my hair to the colors in my clothes.

When I turned five, my hair ceased to be as curly and started to become more textured and extremely thick. The time it took to do my hair increased as the months went on. My mother, sick and tired of how long it took to simply comb my hair, turned to the "white crack," as we called it. I received my first relaxer at the age of six. My mother looked at it as a last resort because my hair was "too uncontrollable." Unfortunately for me, she had never given or received a relaxer before. A relaxer can be a woman's best friend if she's looking to straighten out her natural hair—or her biggest enemy if she's left it in too long. As my mother proceeded to wash out the relaxer, my hair (along with the white chemicals!) went down the drain.

> A relaxer can be a woman's best friend if she's looking to straighten out her natural hair—or her biggest enemy if she's left it in too long.

Years went on, and my hair continued to grow—until my parents got a divorce and my father gained primary custody. We moved to multiple small towns where the number of African-Americans could be counted on two hands, my family included. In elementary school, I had my first experience with the repetitive questions "Why does your hair look like that?" and "How did your hair get like that?"—like there was something wrong with me. These unaware children were my friends, so I didn't see any harm; I became the "educator" on black hair to my curious classmates. When I told them I washed my hair once every two weeks, their faces cringed. They didn't understand how I could stand to have all of that oil in my hair, so I had to explain to them that my hair needed the oil, while theirs would just became greasy. For such a long time I hated my hair because it never looked like the hair of girls in movies or on television shows. I knew for a fact I couldn't make it look like a white girl's hair, but even the girls on the T.V. show "Sister, Sister" had an unattainable hair type.

By the time my mother let me wear my hair straightened on a regular basis, I was a freshman in high school. I loved wearing it down because it made me look older and more mature, and that is what any fourteen-year-old girl wants! I wore it down so much that it started to become damaged and brittle. All of those years of having it in braids in elementary school and letting

> I became the "educator" on black hair to my curious classmates.

it grow went down the drain—just like when my mother had relaxed my hair. Now, as I transition to college, my hair may not be as long as it once was, but I can honestly say that I love my hair. From the length to the thickness to the versatility of it, I love my hair. All of the things I have been through with my hair have made me grow as a person, learn about self-confidence and self-discipline, and realize that hair will grow back. Not only is a woman's hair her pride and glory, but it is an aspect of her that grows and changes as she does.

The Dilemma
Christal Clements

YOUNG women are always taught that their hair is their "crown of glory"—yet, in the black community, young women are placed in a dilemma about what society feels is the "proper" way to style their hair.

Not more than eighteen years ago, I was a part of that group. When I was a young girl, my hair was a breath of fresh air. It was long, shiny, soft and, to my mother's relief, easy to manage with a hair brush and a cup of warm water. My mother loved styling my hair, until it came to straightening. Straightening my hair was like straightening the hair of a Newfoundland terrier. Saying that my hair is thick is an understatement. My hair is THIII-ICK! So, there was no apprehension when my mother discovered the quickest way to straighten my hair: the hair relaxer.

My hair was relaxed from elementary school to high school, and during that time, I experienced severe hair breakage. I was devastated. My long hair was shortened in a matter of seconds. After the experience, I realized I didn't want to place any more chemicals in my hair; I wanted to go natural. There was only one problem—my mother's constant reminders about the frequent payments she had made for the "reconstruction and replenishment" of my hair. Even when I entered college in 2007, I was hindered by her grasp on my hair. I continued to get relaxers.

Initially, I was a low-maintenance person—so my hair was up in a ponytail all the time. Yes, a *ponytail*: one of the most elementary hairstyles a college woman could wear. Fortunately for me, that ponytail helped me meet the love of my life. He loved my long hair, as do most men; however, the desire to go natural lingered in my mind. In December of 2009, I overcame my mother's grasp, and I personally decided to stop receiving relaxers. It was a liberating moment. I didn't have to worry about avoiding certain activities to prevent "sweating out my relaxer." There would be no more scalp burns. I didn't have to run to get out of the rain, and

> My mother loved styling my hair, until it came to straightening. Straightening my hair was like straightening the hair of a Newfoundland terrier.

most importantly, I would have more money to pay for groceries and other necessities because being a college student is rough! So here I am today, going natural.

I was afraid to cut my hair at first, so I decided to slowly grow out the relaxer. At first, the process went smoothly, but soon the hassles began. My hair grows extremely fast, so it wasn't long before I had inches of new growth ending in silky worms of relaxed hair. It drove me nuts! That summer, I decided to cut it off and do the Big Chop. I haven't looked back! I started off with a medium-size Afro—and boy, I'd never felt more confident in my life! I was truly a natural beauty. My whole demeanor changed! I received compliments from people I had never talked to in my life, and my boyfriend, although he disliked it initially, decided he loved my new look, too. My confidence continued to swell.

Later that year, I decided to start dreadlocks. Dreadlocks were always an intriguing hairstyle to me, and I knew the style would fit my laid-back and tranquil personality perfectly. So, there you have it—my crown of glory's journey from soft and shiny to short and damaged to revitalized and replenished to natural and lovely and, finally, to locked and fabulous. It certainly has been a rollercoaster of interesting experiences for me.

Bold and Beautiful
Monet Abrams

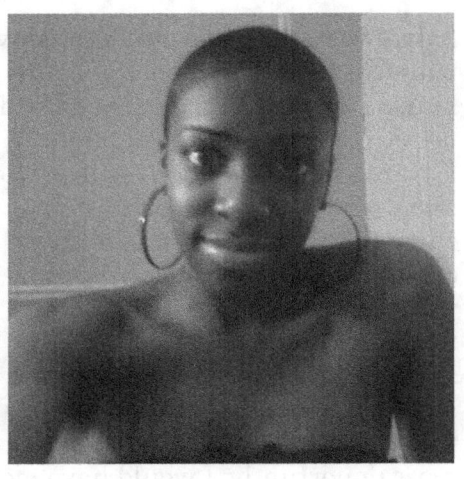

Y ou know how when most people first try new things they are scared or terrified? Well—I am not. The first time I cut my own hair, I was turning sixteen years old. I was already a natural at rinsing and dyeing my hair to change its color, but actually taking scissors and cutting off my hair was something different.

My first hairstyle was black, short in the back, with mini curls on the sides going toward the front and with the middle flipped up. I was so happy that the new look fit my face, and my friends and family were very surprised that I'd actually cut my own hair. I'd had long hair down my back when I was little, although everything went downhill when I got my first perm and started straightening it and braiding my hair.

Compliments were pouring in left and right on my hairstyles; over time, the hairstyles had me looking older and more mature. Little by little, I started getting into more demanding hairstyles such as shaving off my hair on the sides to make a Mohawk. These styles gave me that extra umph to enhance my style. I used to say that I would never put a weave in my hair, but I guess never say never! I started to add blond weaves to my hair, and then I'd change it to red. I didn't put blue or green in my hair because I preferred to color my actual hair in those shades. I took my hair to a whole new level when I shaved off the back and colored my hair orange! Some were shocked that I had the courage to go that far, but most weren't. My grandmother would say that she didn't like my hair *at all* and that I looked "crazy like a clown" and then ask why I would do my hair "like that" (ugly). Criticism is good because you can learn from it to become better. A second opinion is always good, too—but do what you want to do, not what other people say.

There are so many ways to do hair, and I've tried most of them. But even though I've changed my hair many times, I've always stayed true to myself. I'll never change the person I am: the young, vibrant and ambitious Monet. The advice I'd give to someone who wants a hair change is: Be brave, go outside the box, and create your own hairstyle that expresses who you are. Remember that you are living your life for YOU and no one else. Accomplish your dreams, and enjoy life because you only live it once.

> Even though I've changed my hair many times, I've always stayed true to myself. I'll never change the person I am: the young, vibrant and ambitious Monet.

Memories
Shakira Ja'nai Paye

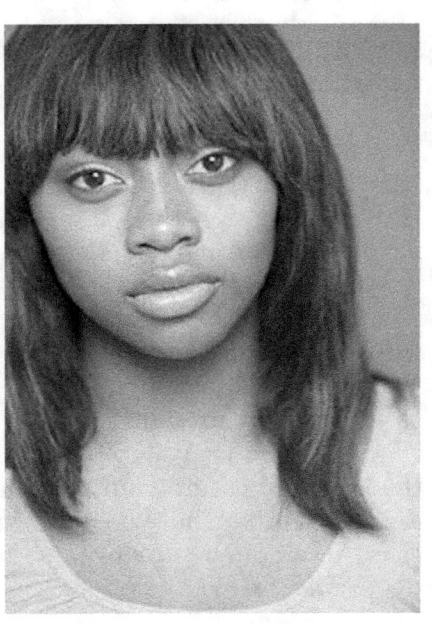

MAYA Angelou says that "hair is a glory you get to share with your family"—and my hair brought me and my mom together to talk about the good, the bad and the ugly. My mom has been my sole hairdresser since I was her little bald-headed baby. She'd always find a hair strand or two to put a big bow on or barrettes around.

My mom went to school for cosmetology and really honed her craft—so you can only imagine some of the styles she tried on my head! Sitting between my mom's legs on our front porch in Baltimore getting braids gave us nothing but time to talk, to laugh and to enjoy hair and each other. I remember when I booked the role of Velma Kelly in my school's production of *Chicago*, I was sitting down getting finger waves done and debating with my mom about how black women *really* wore their hair in that decade. We went on and on, but I Googled it on our computer—and sure enough, I was right! Finger waves were in . . . and maybe bobs were in, too, but I didn't see that picture pop up first.

> Sitting between my mom's legs on our front porch in Baltimore getting braids gave us nothing but time to talk, to laugh and to enjoy hair and each other.

Another hair memory I have was in the third grade when I attempted to prove to my mom that I could do my own hair. I burned my forehead with the curling iron before Picture Day! Thank God my mom knew how to cut a cute bang to cover up my forehead, or I would have looked busted in that picture!

My hair has always been a reflection of my creativity! I used to rock cornrows with beads on the ends during my tomboy/track-and-field days, and during my dance days I wore the oversized hair bun with jewels in my hair. During my senior year, I decided that I wanted blond and pink highlights to reflect my individuality. I think that black hair is the most expressive hair because you can do so much with it. Whether it's straight or twisted, braided or curled, relaxed or kinky, extended or short, black hair is amazing hair. It represents so much about black people: how we are always growing and evolving and how we are all so different. Black hair is full of flavor, just like black people, and that's why I love my black hair!

> I think that black hair is the most expressive hair because you can do so much with it.

Keeping It Short and Sweet
Sabrina Walley

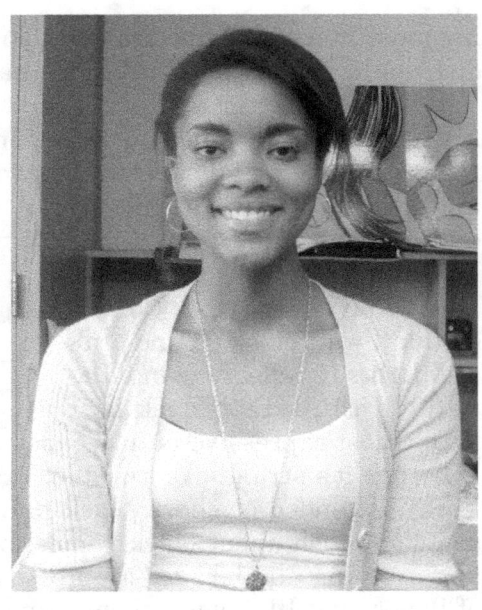

As a child who has grown up with technology advancing every day, I was always glued to the television. And when commercials popped up, the most notable ones, for me, were the hair commercials. Every hair commercial has the generic girl. You'll mostly notice that she's white, with flowing blonde or brunette hair that's silky-smooth. And when she walks down the street, she flips her hair and gives some guy *the look.*

All of this gave me, and probably other girls, the desire to have long, healthy hair. So, in elementary school, my thought was to have hair that extended to the back of my butt. This was mostly because I saw other girls—white girls—with hair that long, and I thought, *Well, why can't I do that?* It wasn't until I reached fifth grade that I knew that it wasn't going to happen. My hair had barely gotten to my shoulders, but it was long enough, and I was okay with that. It was then that I had a serious reality check: My hair was totally different from the hair I admired on T.V. and at school, and for me to have hair that long and healthy would be one heck of a challenge. All of the products that my mom had put in my hair, along with the vast amount of barrettes, were what was keeping my hair shoulder length. The other girls just had to wash it, and it grew shiny, smelled nice and was never oily.

When I reached middle school, I nixed the whole "hair to my butt" thing. When my mom finally let me do my own hair, I started to wash it, blow dry it and straighten it. Every. Day. It wasn't until I had to have my hair cut like one of the Beatles that I realized, *Hey, maybe straightening my hair every day isn't the best idea.*

Because I was so devastated by my hair, my sympathetic mom gave in and let me get braids. Since I had never gotten cornrows before, the pain was unbearable. The digging to keep the cornrows tight to my scalp is something that I'll never forget. My mom washed and braided my hair every two weeks to keep it healthy. Any chance she got during the four hours of braiding, she would chime in and say things like, "You know you can't straighten your hair like that" or "That's too much stress on your hair" or "Do you know how much time I put into your hair to make it that long?" It was as if she were taking my haircut personally. *Um, hello! The hair is attached to MY head. I feel just as much pain as you do.* After two years of braids, my mother and I were tired of them. So, we went to the salon to get my hair relaxed again and hoped that it would not be a disappointment.

> It wasn't until I had to have my hair cut like one of the Beatles that I realized, *Hey, maybe straightening my hair every day isn't the best idea.*

"Your hair is doing really well!" the stylist said.

Oh, thank God. I couldn't take another two years of my mother braiding my hair with her little comments. I'd seriously die. As I walked out of the salon with my new flat, not-oily-or-smelly and long-as-it-could-possibly-be *shiny* hair—I had a little skip in my step! I was confident as could be. Unfortunately, it didn't last for long. By the end of junior high school, the salon lady told me, "Your hair is seriously breaking off, honey. We're going to have to cut it."

Great.

The ratio of tears to cut hair was ridiculous. For every millimeter of hair that was cut, a tear rolled down my face. It just frustrated me! My mother asked how I liked the cut and I simply smiled

> The ratio of tears to cut hair was ridiculous. For every millimeter of hair that was cut, a tear rolled down my face.

and said, "I love it." When we got home, I gently closed my door. I plopped in the bed, put my pillow over my head and cried my frustration away. High school was the same. My oldest sister, who had the best hair of us all, drove me to downtown Philly to get my braids done. Now, at this point I thought the salon was going to be just like my mother, but it was far worse. They shoved the hair into my scalp so much that after they finished (in apparently record time), I had a headache so intense that Advil and Tylenol didn't even work. I went home and lay in my bed—again—crying over my hair. I wanted my own long hair, not artificial hair. Long story short, the same thing happened again: hair grew, was chopped off. Noticing a pattern?

Eventually my senior year rolled around, and I was about to graduate. I walked into the salon with an idea that I thought was my best one yet. *I'm doing this on my own terms. I'm making the decisions.* When I sat down in that chair, I told the stylist, "Leave as much as you want or cut as much as you want. I trust you, and I want something different." She was taken aback, mostly because she knows that both my mother and I like long hair. After about three hours, she spins the chair around and I gaze at my new, short, Rihanna haircut. "I LOVE IT!" I breathed. And this time I meant it with all my heart.

The stylist then went on to explain that shorter hair was easier to maintain and probably most suited for my athletic lifestyle. She also told me something that my other three stylists never did: My hair was breaking off closer to my head, not at the ends or edges. So every time a stylist cut my hair, they weren't cutting where the breakage actually was. As I look back on those seven years of pure *H - E- double hockey sticks*, I think I was secretly being taught a lesson: I didn't need to have long, silky, shiny hair because that wasn't me. Your hair doesn't make you who you are; it's everything else that does.

These Roots
Are Mine
Marggy Charles

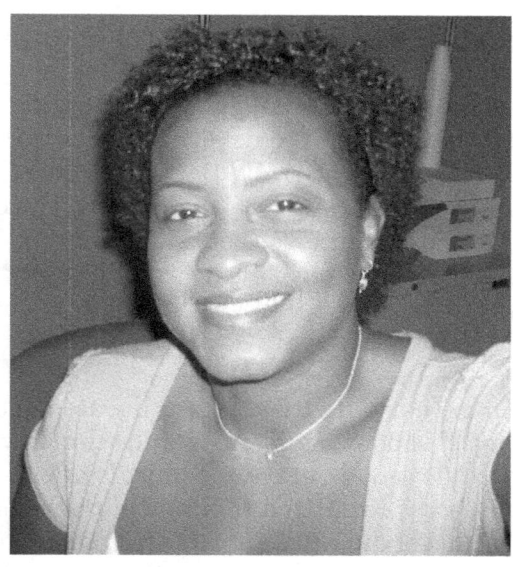

I AM a thirty-eight-
year-old Caribbean/
African-American
woman with natural
hair that is soft, fine and
curly. The story of my
hair changes began in
my preteen years when I
turned twelve years old.
I started wanting to ex-
press my individuality
through my hair, and I paid more attention to which styles best
fit my oval face, my eyes and my lips. I was able to corn braid my
hair and wore my hair in those types of styles every day. When
my aunts noticed that I was losing my hair in the middle of the
back of my head, they warned me to stop combing it the same
way every day. *Did I listen? Not really.* It took some time, but I
eventually stopped and learned a different style.

I got so frustrated that I was one of the only girls in my classroom
that did not have a relaxer. I would pull my hair back into a ponytail and get it hot combed—but that never lasted long. I begged
my mom to give me a relaxer. Of course, she said no, and then we
would fight about it. I was so upset with my mom one day that I
just stopped caring anymore about what I looked like, and so did
she. It was a stalemate until my dad, no doubt tired of looking at
my uncared-for hair, caused my mom to cave in. I got my relaxer,
and it was one of the happiest days of my teenage years.

I kept my hair relaxed for twenty-five years, and I loved it for
so many reasons. The versatility of a relaxed mane is what I
loved. I could make it curly, straight or braided and do a pinup,
French roll, etc. One of my favorite hairstyles with the relaxer
was the shag—I looked so good with that style. I loved parting

it to the side and putting a side bang there so that it had the sultry, elegant look. I would buy my own do-it-yourself relaxer kit at the drug store and go home, relax it, blow dry or wrap it, and sit underneath the dryer for almost an hour and be ready to go. I had the short Halle Berry haircut, the bob and various other layered haircuts with the relaxer. I guess with the relaxed hair I felt accepted by society. I felt normal, and I got more attention from guys. Almost every woman in my family had a relaxer, but my own self-esteem was not where it should have been. Emotionally, I did not really know who I was.

In my early thirties, I was educated enough to start questioning myself about my identity and what I was projecting to others. I would read about how chemicals affected my hair, my health and my body. I realized that one of the reasons I did not work out is because I did not want to sweat out my perm. I realized that I was being a slave to my perm. *Wow!* I would say to myself. *I have to be a deeper person as I get older—not one that conforms to what the world is feeding me or what "they" expect of me.* I found myself getting my hair relaxed less and less often but still could not let it go, even though I knew I needed to make a change.

> I have to be a deeper person as I get older—not one that conforms to what the world is feeding me or what "they" expect of me.

At age thirty-six, I made a decision to start working out again seriously. I registered at the nearest gym and was sweating out my perm every day. I finally decided to go to the barber and cut my hair down to my roots! I felt liberated, brave, confident and natural—*and I still looked good.* I couldn't believe it! I saw that I was not my hair. I was beautiful Marggy.

I'm not defined by my hair; I don't spend enormous amounts of money anymore to make my hair look a certain way. I am happy with my hair now. I sometimes wear it in an Afro or just get it braided like a Nubian sista. When I feel like having straight hair, I wear wigs and love them, too—but the main thing is that my roots are mine, they are natural and I love it.

Hair Care Independence, Granted!

Enongo Lumumba-Kasongo

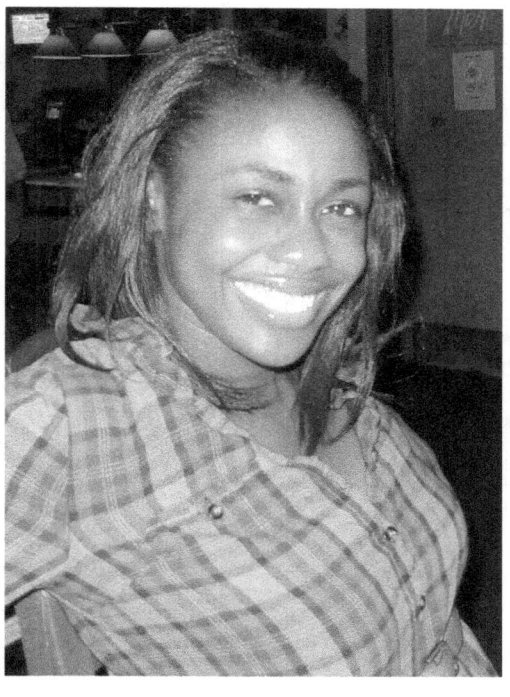

SINCE I was five I had either worn braids or pulled my natural hair into two puffs on the sides of my head. My only experience having my hair relaxed (by my best friend's mother, which resulted in my losing most of it) had sufficiently convinced me that I was never going back. Until, that is, I met a stylist who made me consider changing my life plans solely to preserve my hair.

The summer after I graduated from college, I moved to Houston to work as a teacher through a national teaching program. My roommate, Amber, who was also new to the city, experimented with different hairdressers every week to find someone who could save her relaxed hair from the Houston humidity until she was finally satisfied with a man named Ken. Every time she returned from Ken's salon, I would reflect on my awful experience with relaxed hair and convince myself that it wasn't worth it. As the growth beneath my braids began to show and my head began to itch, though, I thought about how nice it would be to wash and style my hair in a fresh new way every week. Finally, one night I decided to do the unthinkable. I asked Amber for Ken's number and called him to set up an appointment.

That Saturday I arrived at Ken's salon anxiously. As soon as he was finished I jumped out of my seat and stared in the mirror in disbelief. My dark-brown relaxed hair looked lustrous and healthy! Tears came to my eyes as I paid and thanked Ken, immediately setting up my appointment for the following week. As soon as I saw Amber, she squealed with delight and hugged me. On Monday, my students told me I looked like a movie star. Every week at church, members of the congregation would stop to remark and tell me how beautiful my hair always looked. So, without concern for my bank account and out of fear of messing up my trademark, I diligently continued to go back to Ken every week.

> Without concern for my bank account and out of fear of messing up my trademark, I diligently continued to go back to Ken every week.

Eventually my fixation on keeping my hair "perfect" began to dictate my life. I missed important engagements because they overlapped with my hair appointments. I stopped paying my bills on time because I needed the money for Ken. I didn't realize how serious my problem had become until my two-year service in the teaching program came to end. As I talked to Amber about my plans, I realized that I was more anxious about what I was going to do with my hair than what I was going to do with my life! I was completely terrified of my own hair. For the last two years I had been handling it with the utmost care and attention through Ken's excellent service, and I didn't trust anybody, including myself, to wash and style it properly.

I soon realized, however, that I would have to leave Houston because the graduate program I had fallen in love with was in New York. Before I left, though, I asked Ken if he could give me a brief tutorial and purchase for me the products that I would need in order to maintain my hair. On my last Saturday, he provided me with all of the prod-

> My fixation on keeping my hair "perfect" began to dictate my life.

ucts he had used on my hair as well as directions for their use. We hugged briefly, and by the next day I was in New York.

It took me two weeks before I washed my hair for the first time. Following Ken's instructions, I spent two hours washing and styling my hair. As I flatironed the last section, a rush of exhilaration ran through my body. *I was no longer scared of my own hair!* Immediately, I became thankful that my career interests had forced me to leave Houston so that I could redefine my priorities. Of all the things to be scared of in life, I realized that hair should never be one of them.

The Queen Finds Her Voice

Johnene Benson

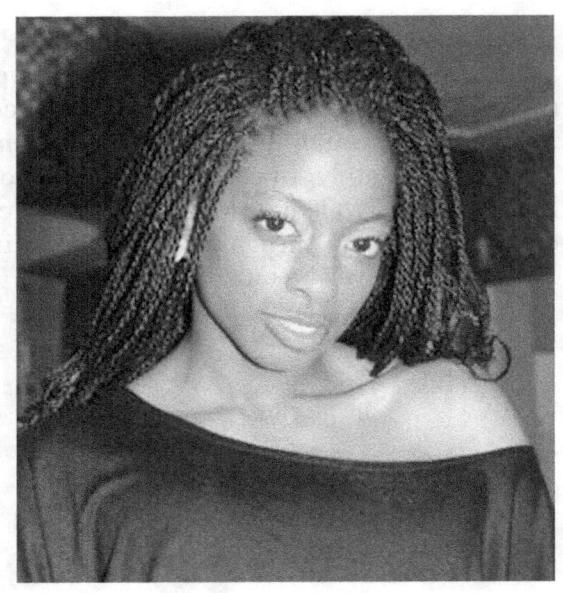

L ET me take you back to the beginning of my freshman year at Winston-Salem State University. At the end of the first week, my orientation leader pulled me aside and told me to apply to be the Homecoming Queen of my class; he felt like I would be a great candidate for the Miss Freshman position. Within a week of the application deadline, all of the qualified Miss Freshman candidates and I were invited to come and chat with the current queens. Toward the end of the meeting, Miss Junior asked if we had any questions. To be honest, I felt like I could handle this position and was ready for this new journey, but I was curious about one thing. "Do the queens always have to wear the same hairstyle?" I asked. "I am natural, and I am not getting a relaxer!" Miss Winston-Salem State University said, "Let's focus on campaigning questions for now."

Sure enough, on September 11, 2009, I became Miss Freshman; over half of my class voted for me! The next day, I had to meet with the other queens, and Miss Sophomore started to chuckle when she realized that I was the girl who had asked the question about hair. We actually met to discuss what we were going to do with our hair for the upcoming football game! With all of the queens having relaxers, I knew a problem would arise since we all had to wear the same hairstyle. When the advisor walked into the meeting, she immediately told me, "Congratulations, and welcome, but I need you to know that you are not going to wear that natural stuff on my court."

As the year went on, Miss WSSU helped me to block out some of the harsh comments of our advisor. As a freshman who was a little insecure when it came to my hair, I was hurt when the advisor disrespected it. Then I grew tired of blowouts, weaves and everyone telling me what I should do, so I gave in. I let two years of being natural go down the drain and allowed my mother to give me a relaxer for Thanksgiving break. I only did this to keep our advisor off of my back and to blend in with the other queens. I was tired of being the burden to the royal court. I wish I would have known that I would later be a burden to my own self.

By the end of January, I needed a touch-up. I asked one of my colleagues if she could relax my hair. She told me that she did not have any more neutralizing shampoo and conditioner, but she had enough relaxer to relax my hair. She used Suave Naturals shampoo and conditioner to substitute for what she did not have in her Motions kit. Nevertheless, when she finished, I went back to my room, swooped my hair in the front and pulled it back into a sock bun. I could never see the back of my head when I did my hair, so when I finished, I would rely on the opinion of my roommate before I ever left our room. My roommate was not in the room when I did my hair, but she walked in just before I was ready to leave, and I showed her my style. When I turned around to see her face, she looked puzzled. I asked her what was wrong, and she took a picture with my cell phone and showed me. I freaked out when I saw that all of my hair in the back was missing! My scalp had felt weird when I was brushing my hair, but I just thought that maybe my head was still tender from the relaxer.

I screamed so loudly that my resident assistant ten doors down heard me. The R.A. flew in, gave me hug and advised me to go to one of her friends on the fourth floor who would help me out. When I got downstairs and took my hair out of the bun, I noticed that all of my edges were starting to fall out as well. When I explained what had happened to the young lady, she told me that I had made a mistake by allowing my friend to use regular shampoo rather than neutralizing shampoo. The neutralizing shampoo prevents the relaxer from eating the hair away.

My scalp was really sore, and my hair was so damaged that wearing wigs was my only solution. I hated those itchy things! I could not believe that I had changed and harmed myself just to please other people. Here I was, the queen of my class, and the confidence that I thought I had to inspire others was gone. No. In fact, it was never there; I had allowed the appearance of my hair to define me. Now that I know better, I am a better woman today. Apparently my classmates could see the difference as well because they voted for me to have the title of Miss Sophomore 2010-2011. Although the moment when I lost my hair made me feel like I had lost my identity, I am grateful that my little tragedy is now my testimony.

It has been a year and seven months since the relaxer disaster, and my hair has grown back healthier than it has ever been. If I had not gone through this life-changing experience, I would still believe that my hair defined me. So many people on my campus have been inspired my story that more than 65 percent of the ladies at Winston-Salem State University are natural. This trend led me to create an organization called My Natural. We aim to encourage college women to understand their self-definition while creating activities that will promote the lifestyle of healthy hair.

> Here I was, the queen of my class, and the confidence that I thought I had to inspire others was gone.

As the founder and president of My Natural, I am excited about the journey to come. Chemical-free is the way to be, and my hair does not define my personality. India Arie's "I Am Not My Hair" constantly plays in my head when people throw out negativity. I am blessed to be a natural girl because God took the time to give each strand of my hair a curl. No matter where my career takes me or what people may say, I am never allowing chemicals to flow my way!

On Lock Judgment
Lester Duverce

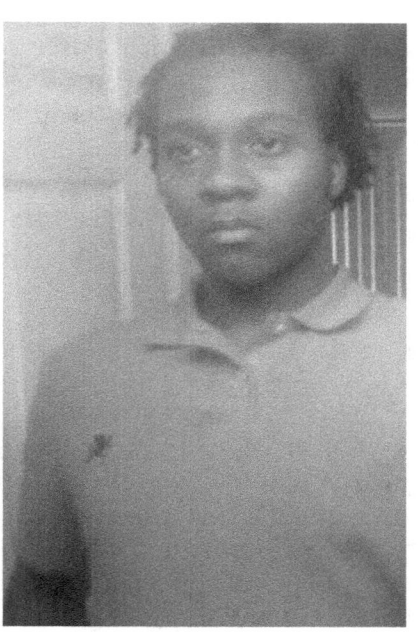

As a young boy, I was always fascinated with dreadlocks, but my parents never allowed my hair to grow past an inch. I would get haircuts every two to three weeks—everything from fades to brush cuts and even waves for a smoother look. At first, I used to think that it was just my parents who did not like locks, but I later found out that it was cultural.

A majority of Haitian parents do not allow young men to wear braids or dreads in their households because it is believed that they will grow up to be rebellious, a future high school dropout or a criminal. Whenever someone with dreadlocks is near, you'll hear negative remarks about that individual. I would often hear things like "Look at those thieves . . .They are bums . . . Men with no education . . . They are nothing but drug dealers, gangsters, thugs" whenever a man with dreads appeared. Other assumptions were that the person must be Rastafarian or smokes weed.

When I turned sixteen years old, I tried to grow my hair. All was well until I got into a small altercation with a few of the kids in my neighborhood. The first thing my parents made me do was cut my hair off. They felt that my hair was the issue, and that simply emulating that style meant that I was looking for trouble. It amazes me how people can view and judge others based upon a hairstyle. I know it is human nature, but who are we to judge others? We are not above or

> It amazes me how people can view and judge others based upon a hairstyle.

superior to anyone else! After graduating high school and moving out of my parents' house, I was finally free to do what I wanted. I wanted to grow locks because I wanted patience, discipline and a way to stand out from others in a positive light. You only live life once, and I wanted to experience having long hair.

> I wanted to grow locks because I wanted patience, discipline and a way to stand out from others in a positive light.

I waited until I turned twenty-one years old to finally grow my hair. I got my first twists ever in January 2011, and my hair was nowhere near long enough to hang on the clips. But I was just delighted to finally have them on my head. I started them off using a comb to twist and black beeswax for hold. Two days later, it was a hot mess. I looked like I had been struck by lightning. (The reason this happened was because I tried to air dry my hair instead of using a real hair dryer to complete the job. It was a valuable lesson learned.) Not giving up hope, I retwisted the locks a week later, using black hair gel and a locking gel. I actually sat under a dryer and got better, longer-lasting results. To some, my hair was nice, neat and waiting to sprout like a plant eager to grow. To others, my hair was hideous, the topic of most conversations and, for many of my friends, the comedy hour.

I would avoid going to certain places just to avoid giving anyone the chance to say something negative. The issue got so bad that a student from school that I had never come across before approached me and demanded that I cut my hair off. A girl even

> A girl even came up to me once on campus and told me that I was "throwing myself away."

came up to me once on campus and told me that I was "throwing myself away." I was basically a laughingstock until the end of spring semester.

Aside from dealing with everyone's negative comments, I had other challenges. Keeping my hair from frizzing, finding someone to retwist the growing dreads and simply not losing a dread were all issues that I faced. (I've already lost a few dreads since

I have been on my journey.) It was also hard to keep my hair clean; that was one of the first lessons I learned when initially growing my locks. My head would get very itchy at times, and whenever I scratched, there would be a lot of flakes. The flakes were brownish gray, sometimes hard and sometimes soft, and always disgusting looking. I was afraid my scalp would eventually dry up and stop my hair from growing. I contemplated cutting my hair on some days. The fact that my hair wasn't all that long caused some individuals to judge me based solely upon my appearance, and they would not take me seriously.

When the month of May came, my hair started growing more. Instead of getting my dreads twisted, I went ahead and interlocked my hair. I also dyed it dark brown. It has been six and a half months since I began my journey, and I really value my hair. There are random times when I want to cut my hair, but I really enjoy the new look. It makes me feel different—wiser and much more mature about many situations. Ever since I started growing my hair, many blessings have come my way. I accomplished a lot of goals, and I got to realize who my true friends really are. My real friends are the ones who gave me encouragement that my hair would grow instead of doubting the new journey I have begun with my hair. Growing my hair makes me strive even harder to achieve my advanced degrees and to become a great entrepreneur in the future—to show everyone that men with dreads can be educated as well.

On Finding My Inner Beauty
Manjit Golden

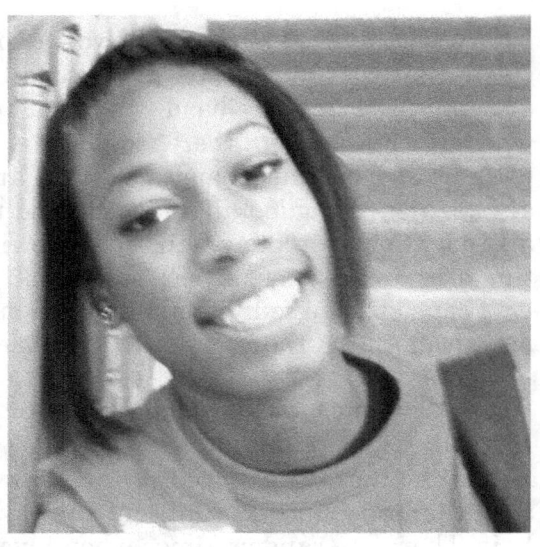

IT seems that all my life, my hair has been a topic of conversation. I was born with a head full of thick, curly hair, but since it only grew down the middle of head, my family jokingly called me Mrs. T. I think I must have gotten that pattern from my mom. My dad always tells me stories about how he fell in love with my mom because of her hair. His stories always start off with "Your mother had the most beautiful head of hair I had ever seen . . ."and end with " . . . but she had a banging body, too." My mom took the best care of my hair when I was little—giving me kiddie perms and flatironing my hair, making it silky and straight. I always received compliments about how beautiful my hair was, and these comments made me feel that I could be as beautiful as my ex-model mother.

When I was very young, I went to school in a small and quiet suburb. There weren't many children of color in my class. Part of the way through second grade, my mom got a new job, and I ended up moving to an urban area in a large city. It was a culture shock, to say the least, since the majority of my class was now African-American. I was a really sweet little girl and had a lot of friends, but there was one girl who hated me, and I could never figure out why. She made up rumors about me, she would push me, and she called me mean names. I never did one mean thing to this girl. I was always the

> It seems that all my life, my hair has been a topic of conversation.

girl who had my hair pressed and straightened and wore cute little dresses—and she was always the girl with the short, nappy braids and jeans with rips in the knees. I would tell my mom how mean the girl was to me, and she'd always tell me that the girl was mean because she was jealous of my pretty hair. Being able to have something that she didn't made me feel like an elitist. I felt better than her. I was thankful that God had blessed me with such a wonderful asset.

When I got into middle school, the questions about my hair began to grow even more. I guess it must be a rarity to be a black girl and have hair down to your waist. Everyone seemed so amazed by it. I have never heard so many theories about why my hair was so pretty. I heard that I was mixed, and that one of my parents was white. I also heard that I had a weave, but I hadn't even heard of weaves by then. I never understood why people were interested in something as dumb as my hair.

Near the end of eighth grade my mom thought that my hair wasn't healthy and that I needed a haircut. I told her that I was tired of having hair that was all one length, and that I wanted it to taper from the front to the back. I don't know how she processed this mentally, because when I looked in the mirror, she had given me the asymmetrical eighties Mary J. Blige haircut. And to make it worse, she had also tried to give me highlights and ended up bleaching the whole top of my head blonde. After a few days, she realized how awful the haircut looked and took me to a hair salon to get it fixed. I went from having this beautiful, long, flowing hair to having hair just above my shoulders. I was devastated at first, but then I went on to realize how insignificant hair really is.

Throughout high school, I had short hair. I realized how much of a hassle long hair was and thought that short hair expressed my personality better. I felt like a bad rocker chick with my shorter spiky hair. And then, that's when it happened. Maybe I listened to India Arie's "I Am Not My Hair" one too many times—or maybe I just lost my mind—because I woke up one morning and decided that I wanted to cut all of my hair off. I went to the salon and told them to cut it into a Mohawk. I felt a rush of adrenaline

> When she was finished, I ran my fingers through it, and for once in my life—*I felt free.*

after the stylist made the first cut. When she was finished, I ran my fingers through it, and for once in my life—*I felt free.* I was finally free from all of the standards of beauty that society had measured and bound me by for so many years. I knew that my new hair was going to change how people thought of me, but I didn't care. My boyfriend wasn't very happy that I had cut my hair off, and he was even less happy when I told him I was going to wear it natural, but he didn't stop loving me because of it. Since then, I have had weaves, braids, extensions and various other hairstyles, but I've realized that it doesn't matter how good my hair looks if I still feel awful on the inside.

The Grass Is Greener— Or Is It?

Natalia Ikheloa

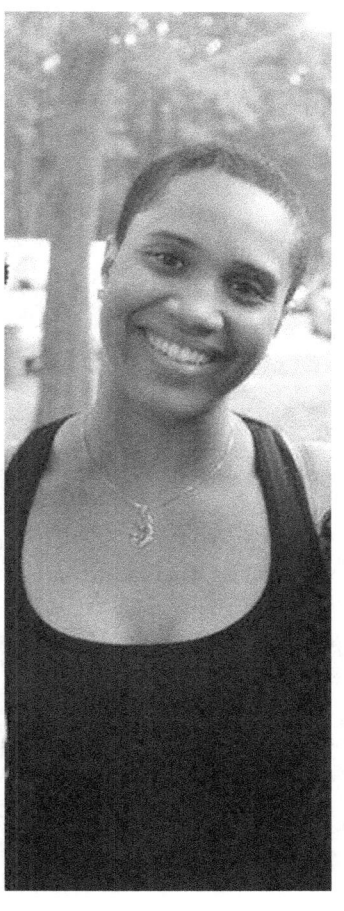

O*UCH!* Another painful experience with my mom attacking the kinks of my thick Nigerian hair.

As far back as I can remember, my hair has always been the most time consuming activity of the day. I often watched in admiration the long, silky hair of Caucasian women that bombarded the television commercials during my youth, wondering why I hadn't taken after my mom's Polish side of the family just a tad bit more. I dreamed of days when my hair would flow effortlessly past my shoulders and not look like an atomic bomb that at any moment might explode. Even the African-American dolls sold in the shops had a texture of hair I'd never thought a person of color could possess.

I often felt terrible about how my mom would painstakingly spend many hours attempting to style the immense amount of hair God had so graciously given me. One fond memory that sticks out in my mind is of the first time she cornrowed my entire head. Predictably, it took approximately twelve hours to complete. My mom gazed at me, smiling at her arduous accomplishment. My brother, who was probably only three or four years old at the time, stared at me and yelled, "That's not my sister!" and ran behind my mother. He truly couldn't comprehend that I was the same person and that only my hair had been altered. I defiantly responded, "Yes, I am, *Papunia*!"—a Polish name I often called him. He slowly walked toward me, examining my new look thoroughly. "You look so different," he uttered in disbelief. As I rushed to the mirror and took in the reflection that was before me, I did something I had never done before until that particular moment—I admired my God-given hair.

Even the African-American dolls sold in the shops had a texture of hair I'd never thought a person of color could possess.

In the eighth grade, while everyone else had relaxed hair, I was still rocking the doo-doo braids and, on rare occasions, cornrows. Somehow my Polish mother got wind of the phenomena of perms—or relaxers, as they are properly called—and suggested getting one. I was determined to find an end to my hair worries and was excited about this new solution to the equation I had attempted to solve for so very long. Skipping alongside my mother, eager to finally obtain this miracle concoction, we walked into Creations Between Us. As I watched the various women that crowded the small beauty salon, a devastating thought crossed my young mind: *What if this miraculous phenomenon didn't work on my hair?* Furthermore, *What if it made my atomic bomb truly explode?* In the span of a second, a glorious occasion became a fretful one. I cautiously walked to the seat I had been instructed to sit in. Waving goodbye to my mom, I spun in the chair and faced the mirror that held the last image I'd have of the hair I had struggled with for so long.

I strolled into the schoolyard as everyone crowded around me, gasping at my new look. Although I wasn't one for attention, the acknowledgment of my peers did bring me a sense of satisfaction. With a new sense of confidence, I was proud to show off my mane, which now looked like those of the women on television that I had admired as a young child. My doo-doo braids were now replaced with ponytails that sat either high or low upon my head.

Although the look of silky hair had been captured, I quickly realized that I still would not be able to wash and go as I had previously imagined. In order to maintain this new look, I now had to ensure that I wrapped my hair before collapsing onto my bed every night, refrain from jumping into any pools and avoid exposing my hair to rain and humid conditions. Let's not forget my new best friend: the hooded hair dryer that I had to sit under for more than an hour at a time. My new hair also became a financial strain because my mother didn't feel quite comfortable applying this chemical to my hair. The effort to maintain my hair in this altered texture may not have been as difficult as before—but the style still demanded a lot of time for upkeep and created a new financial burden.

I'd like to think that I've matured drastically from the youthful perspective I possessed as a child. Instead of attempting to incorporate the traits that have long been viewed as superior, I've learned to embrace my own

> As I watched the various women that crowded the small beauty salon, a devastating thought crossed my young mind: *What if this miraculous phenomenon didn't work on my hair?*

uniqueness and versatility with every curl and kink. It is no longer how society views me that I am concerned with but rather how I view myself. Consequently, I am currently in the process of transitioning my hair back to its original state. Although I am nervous about attacking the atomic bomb again, I am desperately eager to revert to my hair's natural state. This transitioning process will not only alter my hair's state but will also contribute to how I view myself as a woman of color. Today, I welcome and appreciate the many attributes I frowned upon as an ill-informed child. I've come to realize that only in time are we truly able to create our perfect masterpiece, which is the person we fully accept and eventually . . . completely fall in love with.

Ode to the Eighties
Ronchelle Nelson

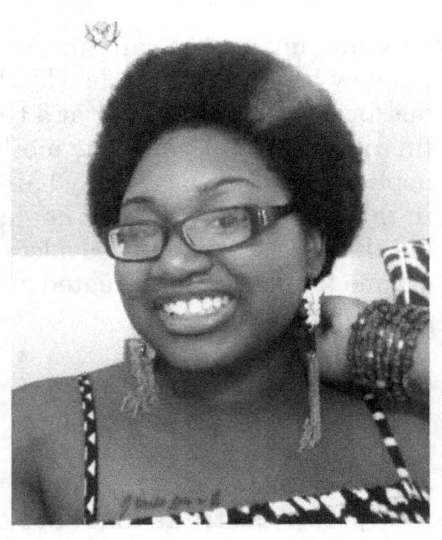

W HEN I first decided to go natural, it wasn't because I wanted to embrace my nappy roots or some other righteous feeling. I went natural because I wanted to look like the girls in the eighties videos. Now, I do not know how I got natural hair from that; all I saw was big hair. I just wanted that massive curly hair that Whitney Houston, Diana Ross, Chaka Khan and the girls from the Full Force videos had. Even though I knew that hair was either a wig or extensions, my mind just told me to go natural.

With this glorious thought, I just stopped perming my hair and combing it in an attempt to get that beautiful hair. Now, the girls in the eighties videos didn't have Afros; they had more of a big curly hair thing going on, and that's what I wanted. I got this crazy idea of paper-bag tying my hair, which is basically me tearing off pieces of a brown bag and rolling my hair with them. This maybe worked once, but then my hair wouldn't even take a curl. I looked a mess. When I look back at pictures of me, I can't even believe I went out like that.

When I first went natural, I did not know there was a thing called transitioning. I just thought that when I stopped perming my hair, I would automatically look like Chaka Khan. Obviously, this did not occur. My hair was brittle and sometimes crazy looking because I did not know how to control my curls or what products to put on them. I finally got fed up and started doing some research.

The first place I went was YouTube. I put "natural hair" into the search engine and started to watch some instructional videos. I saw people using natural hair care products. Users showed videos of their transition and provided others with helpful tips. I was amazed by the numerous ways to style natural hair. I realized that I did not have to wear it out in an Afro all the time. People were dreading, braiding and (the style I feel in love with) twisting. Once I tried it, everything finally came together. Twists were a style that I could use daily. They were a protective style that kept my hair moisturized and healthy.

Anything that wasn't natural I did not want. I had become so against perms, heat and weaves. I just stopped doing all of it. I was happy being nappy, and I wanted all my friends to be natural too. Natural was the way to go, and since my friends saw that, some took out their extensions—but not for long. They needed their creamy crack and *yaky*.

By this time, I had sort of calmed down from my eighties stage, and I really started focusing on getting my hair healthy. Your hair reflects your health. I know I was not the healthiest person (and I'm still not), but we are what we eat, and I didn't want to be a Number 3 Combo with fries and a shake forever. My diet changed. I realized I can't have natural hair if natural food doesn't go inside my body. Drinking more water also was added to my lifestyle because hair dryness could be the effect of not drinking enough water.

> I started a new search for myself, to find that natural girl inside the girl that felt loved, even if no one said it. And to my surprise, she was always there.

Being natural not only changed my diet, but also my way of thinking. I felt like I didn't have to be like everyone else anymore. Fashion, music and everything that was "in style" did not matter to me. I was my own person. I did not look like anyone else around me, so why should I think like them? I started a new search for myself, to find that natural girl inside, the one who wasn't mistreated by the world and had chosen not to conform. The girl that did not need make up, a weave or acrylic to feel beautiful. The girl that felt loved, even if no one said it. And to my surprise, she was always there.

In finding myself, I found truth: truth about the world and, its systems and its governments—and the greatest truth of all, God. In my natural state I've become a better person spiritually, mentally and physically. I am finally at the place where I want to be in life. And when I think back to a year and a half ago and think of all the events that happened in my life when I wasn't natural, it's like I wasn't living my life but the life that my parents had set out for me: the standard way of living that I was accustomed to but not obligated to live by. Things started to come together for me after I went natural. I got out of community college and went to a university. I moved out of my parents' house, got a job and started to provide for myself. As Oprah would say, I'm living my best life.

There's no turning back at this point. I only have two years left until I graduate college. My mind is on the right track, and God is my steering wheel. I love being a natural hair gal; it has changed my life for the better. This is only the beginning of this lifelong journey. Just goes to show that being natural is not just a hairstyle; it's a lifestyle.

And to think it all started with the eighties.

Survivor
Cathy Ervil

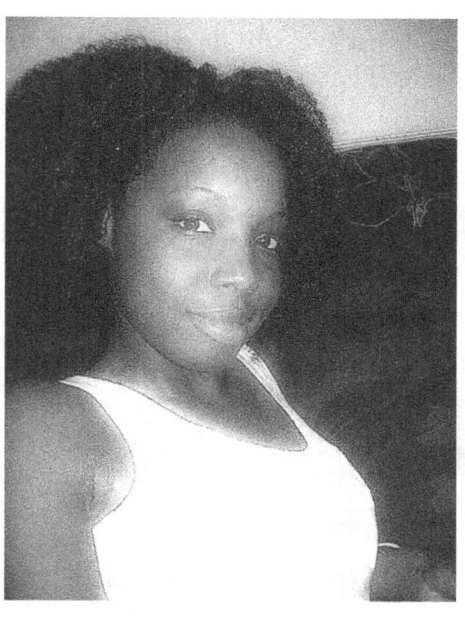

As a twenty-eight-year old African-American female, I have always had kinky, dry, nappy hair—type 4b to be exact. My hair was so nappy that when I was five years old, my mother was so fed up with me crying, *"It hurts!"* that she finally gave me a perm. Every six weeks I religiously got a perm, convinced that I now had "good hair." Getting a perm was like eating: I just had to have it in order to function. However, an unfortunate incident happened that enabled me to discover my hair's true texture and eventually appreciate my uniqueness.

Fast-forward a number of years. I was sitting in my living room savagely eating my bowl of cereal, when all of a sudden I heard what sounded like music to my ears: the faint sound of the mailbox shutting. Eagerly, I ran to the mailbox, and like a mad woman, started looking through the mail until I saw *the golden envelope.* I had received a letter from Florida A & M University stating that I had been officially accepted into the school.

> Getting a perm was like eating: I just had to have it in order to function.

My first semester at FAMU was an academic success; I had a 3.4 grade point average, made the National Dean's List and was admitted into the school of nursing. Nevertheless, about a year and a half later, my joy and happiness came to an abrupt halt. I was diagnosed with Hodgkin's lymphoma—a type of cancer that affects the lymphatic system. I automatically knew that I was going to lose my hair; however, that was the least of my problems. That year I underwent intense chemotherapy, three blood transfusions, two platelet transfusions, a bone marrow transplant and six weeks of radiation therapy.

By the grace of God, I survived and conquered what almost killed me. Finally, after two years of chemotherapy, my hair grew back. That was my first time in twenty years to actually feel and manage my natural hair. As my hair began to grow, I learned to appreciate my kinky, thick and bushy hair. I felt like I was a kid in a candy store; every day I would find different ways to style my newfound hair. Subsequently, I made a life-changing decision: I choose to stay natural. I was tired of the poisonous chemicals that had filled me, and I refused to chemically alter my hair. I am on my fifth year of going natural, and I would not change it for the world. I do have to admit I have been tempted to get a perm because there were days where I couldn't deal with the tangles—but despite my weakness, I've held my ground, and I'm still rocking my kinky hair.

> That was my first time in twenty years to actually feel and manage my natural hair.

Owning My Style
Camille Bridges

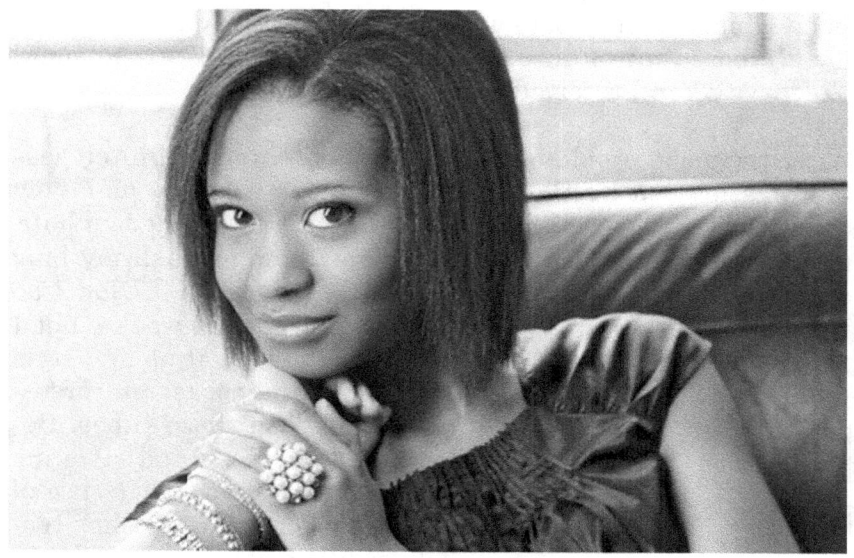

H AIR is the biggest commonality between African-American women. We are judged by our hair length, hair color and overall style. It truly adds to our character and affects our attitude—but how defining *should* hair be?

The style of a woman's hair should not be the attribute that defines or determines her personal success; rather, it should stand as a symbol of her confidence and strength. My hair has not defined me but has changed as my character has changed; I enjoy changing my hairstyles and trying new things.

My childhood memories of the hairdresser include blood, sweat and tears (well, maybe no blood!). When I was about six years old, every two weeks I was forced to sit in a very high chair and allow a woman to blow scorching hot air on my head. She would then run a blazing hot comb through my hair for hours and hours—or what seemed like that long! During each visit, the hairdresser would bring out a bucket to go alongside my chair. I would cry so much—to the point that I would almost begin to throw up. Worse, I might "sweat out" all the hair that had previously been straightened, so that I'd have to get my hair dried and pressed all over again! It was not any different at home. Many times, it was *more* frightening because I had to sit right next to the red stove upon which the hot comb was prepared for my misery. Oh, the joy it brought my mother and hairdresser when I turned eight! This was when I received a perm for the first time.

After the perm, weekly hair appointments were definitely less of a hassle—but I still did not like having someone doing my hair. Over the years, I began learning how to do my own hair, single steps at a time. First, I learned how to wash my hair and later how to blow dry and eventually flatiron it. Now I do it all! My mother still perms my hair every six weeks, but I am able to keep it up and style it (including occasional pressing) between those times. Being able to wash and style my own hair was an early sign of my independence and has truly been a factor in building my self-confidence.

> Many times, it was *more* frightening because I had to sit right next to the red stove upon which the hot comb was prepared for my misery. Oh, the joy it brought my mother and hairdresser when I turned eight! This was when I received a perm for the first time.

When I began to struggle with hair damage and severe breakage when I was fourteen, I knew that it was time to cut my hair. It took me a very long time to do it because I loved having long hair. I was the type who thought it was prettier to have long hair, but the breakage became so bad that I had to cut it. The new style was a bob cut with color, but I honestly thought that I looked like a boy! I assumed that I would be judged because of the haircut, but then I realized that this was just a temporary change in circumstance. I had to adjust and adapt to this new cut. I had to own my new hairstyle. My hairstyle was different from most, but that is just it: I am different. Each and every human being is different from the others around him, so there is no use in trying to change outward appearances to please and be accepted by other people.

I still enjoy doing my hair. It is just another way for me to express who I am as an individual. Maybe my motivation for doing my own hair was encouraged by

> I had to own my new hairstyle.

childhood misery, but the result is independence. Having that control allows me to truly own my hairstyles. I have had my haircut for a few years now, and I absolutely love it. It is not who I am, but it is what I do.

Naturally Proud
Breiana Whittaker

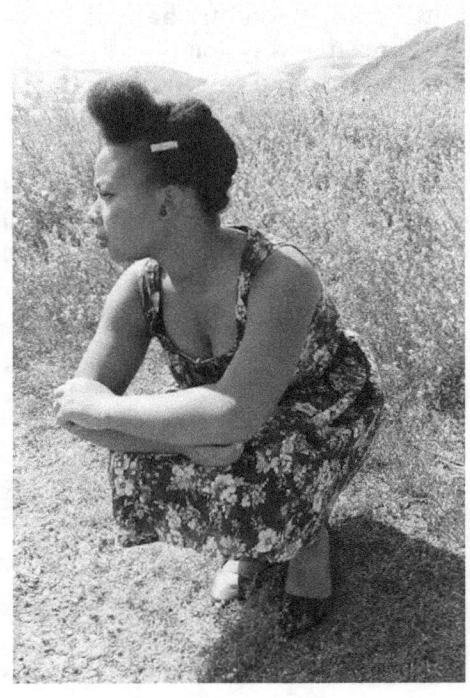

THE first day that I wore my natural hair to school was terrifying. I wore my hair in a bun so that no one could tell that it was not straight anymore. I wore my hair in a bun for a week or two, but I was getting tired of having to *contain* my hair.

One day, I just could not put my hair in a bun any longer. I was fed up. I decided to wear it out in an Afro style. I was so nervous about wearing it to school. The next day, I called my best friends and begged them to walk to school with me to help me boost my confidence. As soon as we stepped onto the campus, I felt all the butterflies.

> Having a natural is not unusual here on the West Coast, but having kinky, tightly coiled curls that defy gravity is something I rarely, if ever, see.

Having a natural is not unusual here on the West Coast, but having kinky, tightly coiled curls that defy gravity is something I rarely, if ever, see. Having my kind of natural hair is just not a popular choice, so I have always worn the "normal" type of hair—which is essentially anything that conceals your natural texture (i.e., weaves, perms, constant straightening, braids or cornrows).

Going to school with natural hair made me feel like I had a giant pimple on my face—except that everyone felt free to comment

132

on it. When I walked into my first class, I immediately regretted my decision to wear the Afro. The majority of the boys in the class were sitting in the walkway, and I had to walk in front of them. They made "Ahhhs" and "Ohhhs," and it felt like an eternity before I finally sat down in my seat. After first period, I had to go to homeroom—with all nine hundred seniors in the gym. As I walked into the gym, my Caucasian and Hispanic friends all gave me positive comments— but when I walked past two black girls, they had nothing nice to say. One said, "Hey Brei, I think my pencil is stuck in your 'fro. I can't find it"; then the other girl said, "Oh my gosh. I have no comment for you Brei . . ." in a very condescending tone. I was so shocked by them. I assumed that my black friends would understand what I was doing, which was going against the norm, but instead they criticized me. I did not let their comments get me down though. I proudly wore my Afro.

> I assumed that my black friends would understand what I was doing, which was going against the norm, but instead they criticized me.

My hair has always been a struggle for me until I grew the confidence to wear my natural hair. Having natural hair for me is so refreshing—it is stronger and thicker and does not just break off like it used to. Having natural hair has been a struggle, but it is well worth it. I am much more confident in myself, and I am just so happy with my hair.

Longing for a Simpler Time
Rebekah Webster

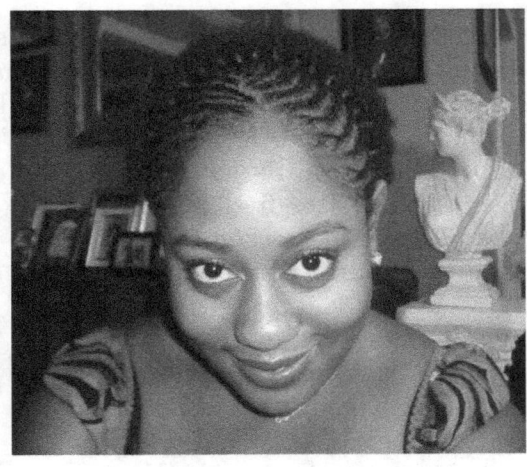

I MISS the nineties, when I did not know a thing about hair, beauty or the newest trends. I miss worrying about when the newest episode of "Rugrats" is coming on and anticipating summer so that I can stay up all night watching all of "The Cosby Show" and "Fresh Prince of Bel-Air" reruns. In those days, there was no time for hair. When you are a child, anything goes. You could slap a ponytail in the middle of your head, and you would still be considered the baddest kid on the block. It did not matter what was on your head.

I had long, curly, thick hair when I was a child. It was beautiful, but I sure did hate when my mother had to "do" it. We broke countless wooden bushes. I was a tender-headed child, and I flinched every time my mother told me to keep my head still.

> When you are a child, anything goes. You could slap a ponytail in the middle of your head, and you would still be considered the baddest kid on the block.

I did not face the pressures of hair until I reached the fifth grade. I thought I was grown and could make decisions for myself, so I was influenced by my older sister to get a relaxer. When I saw her walk out of the Dominican hair salon with her silky, smooth, bouncy black hair, I automatically thought that this would be the cure for my aching knuckles. She did not have to say a word; I was sold on the creamy product, and the relationship would last for years to come.

I believe that most people who have used relaxers must have at least one "bad relaxer" story. In the seventh grade I got a bad relaxer from my aunt that really caused my hair to break off. I was devastated because my hair started falling out, and I had burns all over my scalp. My mother was furious. Although I was upset, too, I was also relieved that I had at least a year for my hair to grow back before I reached high school. I quickly nursed my hair back to health. I continued getting relaxers in high school, so that my hair could be manageable and look good. Do not get me wrong; I was not the girl who had a new hairstyle every week—but hair was still

> When I saw her walk out of the Dominican hair salon with her silky, smooth, bouncy black hair, I automatically thought that this would be the cure for my aching knuckles.

very important to me. In fact, I became obsessed with my hair. It became so bad that I had to ask the teacher to excuse me from class just so that I could make sure that every stand was in the right place! (The proctor did not know that, of course.)

As I began to mature, I decided that I wanted to feel my natural hair again. Initially, I wanted to cut it during my senior year of high school, but between senior breakfast, senior pictures and senior prom, I had too many events that I had to attend. I thought to myself, *I can't be looking like a mess during my senior year of high school!* Honestly, I thought that cutting my hair would make me look like a boy with breasts—at least that's what my father always told me.

I went through two whole years of cutting my hair into styles that I liked for three months, only to end up cutting it all over again. But one day, while cleaning the floors of my dormitory bathroom, I had a sudden epiphany: *I was going to cut off all of my hair, and there was nothing that anyone could do about it!* I had gotten so tired of my hair falling in my eyes while I was trying to scrub the floors. I was done with worrying about sweating out my relaxer, spending money to buy relaxers and going through the long process of washing, blow drying, and flatironing my hair. I was a college student with a $32,000-per-year private-school

I did not see how physically beautiful I am until I cut all of my hair off. I am truly beautiful.

tuition bill who came from a family that is still suffering from the downturn of the economy— and it was time for me to cut off some of that excess spending! I took a pair of office scissors to the front of my hair and did not stop until all I had was peach fuzz on my head.

I did not see how physically beautiful I am until I cut all of my hair off. I am truly beautiful.

Afterword

HAIR aside—in today's global economy, nothing is more important than the relentless pursuit of education. This ideal could not have been more impressed upon my life than by the time that I saw my eighty-year-old grandfather receive his college degree. This one act, perhaps heightened by its seemingly late execution, had a resounding impact on me. This man whose own great-grandparents had been slaves, who'd been born at a time when education for men and women of color was a lofty goal and who'd braved the sorrows of the civil rights movement in the deep Louisiana south still found a way to execute and accomplish his dreams of higher education. No one would have ever blamed him for not completing his studies, given his life struggles, age and relative career success without the degree— but he persevered. He was no prodigy or intellectual genius, but he lived a meaningful life that inspired and continues to inspire. He did not rely on outside expectation or motivation to drive his ambition; he simply held *himself* to a higher standard.

This hands-on lesson in perseverance caused many of us who lived within his realm of influence to consider—or shall I say *reconsider*—ourselves. Our excuses for not achieving one goal or another, educational or otherwise, suddenly lost their power and logic. My grandfather's love for education and achievement instilled in me two very important lessons that I carry forward today in everything I do. The lessons? *Use your talents, gifts and influence (no matter how small or insignificant they appear) to better the lives of those around you, and whatever you start—execute it like there is no tomorrow.*

Our goal through The Science of Black Hair Forum Scholarship Program is to help others reach and attain the highest educational and entrepreneurial heights possible. Proceeds from sales of *The Science of Black Hair,* personal donations and membership subscriptions are used to sponsor our scholarships, giveaways and promotions. For more information on The Science of Black Hair Forum, please visit us on the web at www.blackhairscience.com or www.blackhairscience.com/forum.

Audrey Sivasothy,
author, publisher, and
founder of The Science of
Black Hair Forum

SHARE WITH US

WE would love to hear your reactions to the essays included in this anthology. Let us know which stories you loved (or hated!) and how they've affected you.

We invite you to send us your short essays and stories that you would like to see published in future editions of *Reflections*.

Send submissions to:

ATTN: Reflections Editor
Saja Publishing Company
P.O. Box 2383
Stafford, Texas 77497
www.sajapublishing.com

www.ingramcontent.com/pod-product-compliance
Lightning Source LLC
Chambersburg PA
CBHW070553180626
46817CB00005B/1827